VAGUS NERVE
STIMULATION

Learn the Secrets and Power of Your Nervous System

(Access the Power of the Vagus Nerve With Self-help Exercises)

Grace Johnson

Published by Tomas Edwards

Vagus Nerve Stimulation: Learn the Secrets and Power of Your Nervous System (Access the Power of the Vagus Nerve With Self-help Exercises)

ISBN 978-1-990373-43-5

Legal & Disclaimer

The information contained in this book is not designed to replace or take the place of any form of medicine or professional medical advice. The information in this book has been provided for educational and entertainment purposes only.

The information contained in this book has been compiled from sources deemed reliable, and it is accurate to the best of the Author's knowledge; however, the Author cannot guarantee its accuracy and validity and cannot be held liable for any errors or omissions. Changes are periodically made to this book. You must consult your doctor or get professional medical advice before using any of the suggested remedies, techniques, or information in this book.

Upon using the information contained in this book, you agree to hold harmless the Author from and against any damages, costs, and expenses, including any legal fees potentially resulting from the application of any of the information provided by this guide. This disclaimer applies to any damages or injury caused by the use and application, whether directly or indirectly, of any advice or information presented, whether for breach of contract, tort, negligence, personal injury, criminal intent, or under any other cause of action.

You agree to accept all risks of using the information presented inside this book. You need to consult a professional medical practitioner in order to ensure you are both able and healthy enough to participate in this program.

Table of Contents

Introduction

Several processes throughout your entire body are controlled by the autonomic nervous system—the system responsible for automatic regulation. These are processes such as digestion, breathing, and regulating your heart. This is where your vagus nerve comes into play. The vagus nerve is effectively a loop through which the brain is able to communicate with the body, and then the body is able to send feedback back to the brain by continuing along with the loop.

This means that your vagus nerve is absolutely critical in bodily regulation. If it is not functioning properly, then the rest of the body suffers from all sorts of other consequences as well. This means that the most important information to functioning properly is going to be routed through the vagus nerve, and if the vagus nerve cannot properly push it through, whether due to being either too active or not active enough, it will wreak havoc on your body.

As you read through this book, you will learn all about this process. You will learn about why the vagus nerve is so critically important to your own biological functioning. You will learn about how it is directly related to several of the most important functions of your body and how it is imperative in nearly every single aspect of your life. You will learn how everything can go wrong with even minor disruptions to the nerve's ability to function, and you will learn how to combat it.

In particular, you will address several common ailments—you will learn about how the vagus nerve impacts chronic illness, PTSD, anxiety, inflammation, depression, and even anger. As you read through these chapters, you will learn about how the vagus nerve's malfunctioning is related to each of these issues, and also how you can help mitigate these issues through activating the vagus nerve. Lastly, you will be given two exercises to activate the vagus nerve per chapter.

There are plenty of books on this subject on the market, thanks again for choosing this one! Every effort was made to ensure it is full of as much useful information as possible; please enjoy!

Chapter 1: The Polyvagal Theory

Customarily the autonomic nervous system was perceived for its guideline of the different instinctive "programmed" capacities, for example, absorption, breath, sex drive, propagation, and so on. The old model of pressure or-unwinding depended on perceiving just two circuits— the sympathetic and the parasympathetic. In the old model, the sympathetic nervous system was viewed as dynamic in stress reaction to dangers and risk. The parasympathetic nervous system, on the other hand, communicated in the unwinding reaction and was related with the capacity of the vagus nerve. This more established, all around acknowledged model of the autonomic nervous system expected that there is a solitary vagus nerve, and it didn't assess the way that there are really two very unique neural pathways that are both called "vagus."

The Polyvagal Theory starts by perceiving that the vagus nerve has two separate branches—two discrete, particular vagal nerves that begin in two unique areas. We get a progressively exact portrayal of the operations of the autonomic nervous system on the off chance that we think about that the autonomic nervous system comprises of three neural circuits: the ventral branch of the vagus nerve (positive states of unwinding and social engagement), the spinal sympathetic chain (battle or flight), and the dorsal branch of the vagus nerve (slowdown, shutdown, and burdensome conduct). These three circuits direct our substantial capacities so as to assist us with looking after homeostasis.

The Polyvagal Theory likewise displays another measurement to our comprehension of the autonomic nervous system. The autonomic nervous system not just controls the capacity of our inward organs; these three circuits additionally identify with our emotional states, which thusly drive our conduct. Individuals who give massage know for a fact that one individual's body may be excessively tight, another may be excessively delicate, and a third can feel "perfectly." Usually, when specialists are prepared to give massage, they figure out how to discharge pressure in a strained muscle. Notwithstanding, this methodology doesn't take a shot at a body that needs adequate tone.

Movement bolstered by the spinal sympathetic chain empowers us to battle so as to meet a danger or flee so as to maintain a strategic distance from it. This is on the grounds that hard, tense muscles allow us to move the whole body all the more rapidly. Worse hypertension is additionally expected to get the flow of blood into muscles that are strained and hard.

Low levels of muscle tonus are discovered when the dorsal vagal circuit is actuated when there is no compelling reason to tense the muscles to battle or escape (or, at times of outrageous threat, when the body's endurance reaction is to close down). Low blood pressure is adequate to get the blood into delicate, limp muscles. In its outrageous structure, this low blood pressure may make individuals lose cognizance and swoon. The restorative term for this is "syncope." Normal blood pressure is suitable for muscles that are neither tense nor limp—muscles that vibe without flaw. In states of social engagement, there is commonly no risk or threat in our condition or body. Our nervous system enrolls this reality, so we don't need to do anything; we can genuinely unwind and appreciate being with others. As far as the Polyvagal Theory, we can be immobilized unafraid, outrage, or burdensome action when we are in a condition of social engagement. Our blood pressure, blood sugar, and temperature are generally typical. We can stay composed yet wakeful and alert.

A handshake gives us a decent sign of the condition of someone else's autonomic nervous system. An excessively tight body, as a rule, results from an incessant condition of action in the spinal sympathetic chain, where the whole solid system is ceaselessly arranged to battle or escape. Such an individual typically has an excessively compelling handshake, pressing more earnestly than would normally be appropriate. The inverse is valid for somebody lacking strong tonus— generally an indication of over-movement in the dorsal vagal circuit. This individual, by and large, has a limp, moist, and now and then chilly handshake. In the event that our handshake is perfect, it is the ventral branch of the vagus nerve that is transcendent. We may have a few pressures in individual muscles. However, the strained muscles loosen up rapidly, and a massage specialist will see that our body likewise feels right. The tonus of the muscles is just one of numerous approaches to screen the condition of the body's nervous system.

Chapter 2: The Relation between the Vagus Nerve and Mental Health

Your Vagus Nerve and Mental Health

Did you know your vagus nerve plays a part in your mental health as well? It isn't just a physical sensation but also a mental sensation. Sure, the fatigue and exhaustion are physical, but psychiatric conditions are affected by your vagus nerve, we'll highlight just what they are, and how to properly understand the connection between your vagus nerve, and your mental health.

Your vagus nerve is a nerve that is connected to not only your brain and heart but to pretty much every upper body function.

The vagal tone you experience changes over time and vagal tone is a natural biological process within the vagus nerve.

When your vagal tone is high and proper but means you're relaxing from the stressful situation and calming down.

But your vagal tone plays a part in your emotions, and how your physical health happens. If your vagal tone is higher, then your physical and mental health will be higher too.

Your vagal tone and vagal response naturally reduce stress. Stress can make you experience both positive and negative emotions. A little bit of stress is healthy, but you should always respond to it after the stressful situation by calming down, but that's not always the case. Your vagal tone changes the brain's responses, stimulates the digestion of the body, and in general helps to relax.

Relaxing is good for the body if you're always stressed, you'll have trouble doing many things. Too much stress isn't good for you.

When we're too stressed

Having too much stress isn't a good thing. Stress makes you depressed, anxious, and also angry, and it can affect your ability to make rational decisions, whether it's in daily life, or the long run.

It also affects your dopamine and serotonin levels, both of which are neurotransmitters that handle our mood. Your vagus nerve handles the variability of this whenever it can, and when you're relaxed, you have more dopamine, serotonin, and you'll feel better.

For many of us, stress is a healthy way to accomplish things, but with the way life can be, it can be almost too much in many cases, and vagal tone is affected when we're stressed.

When you feel stressed, depressed, or anxious, your vagal tone changes, and oftentimes, you're more focused on negative emotions, and psychiatric conditions. Epilepsy also increases when your vagus nerve isn't properly stimulated.

You can measure this in different ways by looking at the EmWave2 waves which measure your heart rate variability, which shows your vagal tone too.

Higher vagal tone means everything is working better, and it can also help to stimulate your vagus nerve. You'll notice that when your vagus nerve is properly stimulated, you also respond to situations more positively, whether it is emotional, or physiological situations. Your brain and emotions are properly connected, and it can help offset the issues that mental illness provides to you.

Your vagus nerve is the connection between your digestive system, brain, and other conditions. It also controls inflammation too. But, your vagus nerve also handles mental health conditions, and there are many that your vagus nerve is attributed to.

What Conditions does a low vagal tone cause?

Low vagal tone or otherwise known as your vagus nerve isn't properly stimulated, because many different conditions in the body and some of them are significant. Besides anxiety disorders and depression, it also is found in other types of conditions too.

Degenerative mental health conditions, such as Alzheimer's and dementia, were found to be connected to your vagal tone. That's because, the inflammatory response in the brain isn't curbed, which causes degeneration of the nerve cells, and thereby this condition.

Migraines and other problems in the head, including tinnitus, are also attributed to your vagus nerve. When it comes to tinnitus, it's because your vagus nerve is very close to where your ear is and wraps partially around the inner parts of the ear.

But, it's more than just these conditions. Addictions, eating disorders, personality disorders, even autism spectrum conditions are oftentimes attributed to your vagus nerve. That's because the mental health effects that come about due to the physical problems this possesses can play a major role in your body's' ability to handle this.

Drug and alcohol addiction oftentimes happen because of this. It's because when the vagal tone isn't fully activated, it causes the body to seek out other alternatives since it's not getting enough serotonin in the body. For addicts, the happy feeling they get when they shoot up or take drugs, helps with this and can make them feel good, but it doesn't fix the problem of the vagus nerve not being stimulated, and oftentimes, it makes the problem worse.

But it isn't just serious conditions. Poor memory, mood swings and even mood disorders, MS, OCD, and several mental diseases and mental conditions can oftentimes come about because of this.

Chronic fatigue is another problem too, and we'll get to that in just a moment.

Chronic Fatigue and Your Vagus Nerve

Your vagus nerve controls how your body handles certain conditions. When it's overstimulated, your body is fighting with the sympathetic nervous system, which is always putting you on high alert. But, if you're always on high alert, it'll make you feel third and fatigued all the time.

This isn't just temporary tiredness either, it's oftentimes a serious condition, where you feel fatigued no matter what you do and no matter how hard you try, and it doesn't go away. This can be attributed partially to digestive and nerve health, but it does tie into the vagus nerve.

So yes, chronic fatigue is caused by your vagus nerve, and it can make things very hard on you. It's also due to the breathing you're doing, because many people who have trouble breathing oftentimes suffer from the improper vagal tone, and that's because people don't realize how impactful this can be on the body.

Brain Injuries

Having a vagal tone that isn't properly stimulated does affect your brain and how it works. When your vagus nerve isn't properly stimulated, allowing you to get that air you so desperately need, your body won't get enough oxygen. Oftentimes, this causes vagal syncope, which is fainting involuntarily. If you're not careful, you'll faint in a location that isn't ideal, which then causes head and brain injury. Sometimes, this trauma can be so bad that you can't do anything about it, and instead, you're unable to perform functions in life.

This is probably the worst it can get, but it can negatively affect the rest of your body, even your life if you're not careful.

This is usually a more serious situation, but it's still worth mentioning, because many don't take into consideration what might happen if your vagus nerve isn't stimulated properly, and the truth is, a lot can happen if it's not, so remember that.

Vagal tone and Mental Health

Your vagal tone is part of your mental health, and a healthy vagal tone means better mental health. You can reduce inflammation, negative feelings, and loneliness, even your instances of heart attacks or stroke if you're not careful.

Many people who have a higher vagal tone as part of a feedback loop between these emotions are oftentimes happier and in better physical health.

Healthy vagal tone also affects your social conditions too. You want to talk to other ore, and don't feel held back by depression and sadness when you have healthier vagal tone. You'll notice that you're much better off if you take care of your vagal tone, and you'll notice that your vagal tone will improve your social interactions.

Humans are social creatures. We need to speak to others for the most part, or else loneliness sets in. we try to fill that void as much as we can, and even introverts need someone to talk to now and then. Your vagal tone improves when discussing subjects with others, or just simply speaking in order to generate emotions.

When you're in a good mood, and your vagal tone is healthy, you'll notice that you have better human communications, and your bonds with others become more close-knit. That's because, you're taking care of your vagal tone, and are working to improve your vagus nerve stimulation.

Your vagus nerve does tell you about the "gut feelings" and the anxiety and fear that you feel within the brain, and stress and depression are regulated via the vagus nerve, and your immune system plays a part as well. When there are more cytokines in the body, you'll have better immunity, a happier body, and puts you're a less risk for mental health conditions.

Cytokines also help with some types of depression, especially those with low mood, low motivation, and low energy. If you have more control over this, you'll feel better too.

What can we do About This?

While you can't just "turn off" mental health conditions, stimulating your vagus nerve will help with this. By properly breathing, and taking the steps to calm the body down, it can help curb anxiety disorders and stress-related to anxiety. It will help improve your mood.

Even just working with socialization can help with stimulation your vagus nerve. Communication has been proven to help with your vagus nerve, a properly stimulating it via communication will aid you in bettering your vagus nerve.

Chapter 3: The Peripheral Nervous System

At the outset of this book, we focused on the CNS. The CNS is the essential unit that controls the functioning of the entire nervous system. As we have also established, the CNS plays a pivotal role in ensuring that the body is able to sustain life, repair itself and go about daily chores and activities.

At this point, we are going dive into the Peripheral Nervous System (PNS). The PNS is responsible for a myriad of functions and activities. Hence, it is just as important as the CNS, though with a more specialized task.

The PNS is made up of two main components: the somatic nervous system (SNS) and the autonomic nervous system (ANS). Each one of these individual nervous systems provides specific functions to the CNS. As such, they are significant insofar as providing the brain with the information it requires on the movements of the body and essential biological functions.

The Somatic Nervous System

The SNS has a very specific task, that is, to relay information from the limbs to the CNS. The SNS is made up of a network of nervous fibers that allow the brain to control the movement of the limbs. This is what enables walking, sitting, typing, eating, playing sports and so on. Without this network, the brain would be unable to control voluntary movement. Therefore, a person would not be able to move voluntary. Since this is not the case, we can only speculate as to how the body would be controlled.

The SNS controls muscles and their movements through a series of voluntary responses, either stemming from an individual's desire to carry out a specific activity, or as a result of the response which emanates from an external stimulus.

Consider this example:

First, an individual wants to grab an apple. This is a voluntary movement that requires the brain to signal the limbs (arms and hands) to reach out and grab the apple.

Next, the brain receives input from a visual stimulus. The brain has perceived there is a fire. As such, the brain sends a signal to the legs to get moving and hightail away from the fire. In this case, this is a matter of responding to the external stimulus.

Now, it should be noted that the reaction to the fire is part of the ANS, it is worth mentioning that without the SNS, the legs would be unable to make any kind of movement whatsoever. So, the SNS plays a crucial role in survival.

The Autonomic Nervous System

The ANS is incredibly important in the body's sustainment of life. Without it, the essential biological functions, the involuntary kind, would be impossible to carry out. After all, imagine how hard life would be if you have to remember to keep breathing or make a conscious decision to digest food.

As such, the ANS is commonly associated with biological functions that are broken up into two main categories: the sympathetic nervous system and the parasympathetic nervous system.

The Sympathetic Nervous System

The Sympathetic Nervous System is associated with the fight-or-flight response that virtually all living beings have. In humans, this is a response to an external stimulus. In the example of the fire, the reaction to the perceived threat is generated by the Sympathetic Nervous System. This system sends a signal to the

CNS which then sends an order to the SNS to get moving.

Also, the Sympathetic Nervous System is considered to be on stand-by and comes into action generally when levels of stress increase. The hormone known as cortisol plays a key role in this situation. When the body detects higher levels of cortisol, the Sympathetic Nervous System kicks into gear.

Here are the main attributes of the sympathetic nervous system:

The bronchioles in the lungs are expanded to permit more air into the lungs, which build the oxygenation of the blood and stay aware of the increased blood flow through the lungs as a result of the expanded heart rate.

Bladder and sphincter control. This part of the nervous system is associated with bladder and sphincter control at a conscious level. In fact, loss of control of these two functions can be traced back to some kind of damage in this biological function. As a result, care needs to be taken to avoid any potential issues with these functions.

The pupils of the eyes become dilated. Since the sympathetic nervous system is regularly enacted when individuals are under stimulation, the dilation of eye pupils is a clear sign of some type of increase in the nervous system's response to the stimulus in question.

Increased heart rate. When the heart increases, whether as a result of physical exertion or a stress response, the flow of blood increases thereby leading to greater amounts of oxygen flowing through the body.

The digestive system is slowed as a result of the increased response to stress, among other biological functions which are slowed down. This slowdown is the result of the body's need to prioritize resources with regard to the physiological response that is in course.

The adrenal organs epinephrine and norepinephrine. The adrenals are a couple of hormone-creating glands situated over the kidneys that react to stress. Together, the epinephrine and norepinephrine discharged by the adrenal glands have an essential impact on the sympathetic nervous system by increasing heart rate, expanding the bronchioles, and increasing glucose discharge from the liver. Moreover, norepinephrine is likewise known to increase alertness. It might appear to be repetitive that these hormones have indistinguishable activities from the sympathetic neurons, however, hormones have longer enduring impacts than nerve driving forces, so while the underlying battle or flight reaction is interceded by neurons, these hormones serve to fortify and support the reaction.

The liver discharges glucose into the circulatory system giving the body an increased caloric supply that will be prepared to control the muscles in the event that it is required.

The Parasympathetic Nervous System

The Parasympathetic Nervous System plays an active role insofar as keeping essential bodily functions moving. As such, the parasympathetic nervous system is commonly called the "feed and breed" system since it controls common procedures that are indispensable for the sustainability of ordinary life. The elements of this system include lowering pulse and heart rate after a spike of the fight-or-flight reaction, regulation of stress hormones such as cortisol and the blood pressure control in addition to biological functions such as breathing, circulation, digestion and sensory management.

Parasympathetic nerves begin in the spine, emerging from the spinal nerves of the central nervous system. The axons of this system are generally very long and stretch out into ganglia throughout the remainder of the body. These ganglia are commonly situated in, or close to, organs, enabling the parasympathetic nervous system to quickly send and receive messages from all over the body. Since the parasympathetic nervous system starts in the spine, it does not ordinarily require conscious thought to activate its functions.

The parasympathetic nervous system begins from average medullary locales (core vague, core tractus solitarius, and dorsal motor core) and is regulated by the nerve center. Vagal efferents reach out from the medulla to postganglionic nerves that innervate the atria by means of ganglia situated in cardiovascular fat cushions with neurotransmission that is adjusted through nicotinic receptors. Postganglionic parasympathetic and sympathetic cholinergic nerves at that point influence heart muscarinic receptors.

Parasympathetic enactment can influence atrioventricular nodal conduction intervened prevalently through the left vagus nerve. Besides, muscarinic receptors on vein dividers can cause vasorelaxation through nitric oxide (NO), regulated pathway however can likewise cause vasoconstriction by legitimately enacting smooth muscle. Subsequently, in spite of the fact that the sympathetic nervous system affects cardiovascular physiology in an all-or-none kind of reaction, the parasympathetic nervous system can have a specific balance at different levels.

Vagus nerve afferent actuation, beginning incidentally, can adjust efferent sympathetic and parasympathetic capacity centrally and at the degree of the baroreceptor.

Efferent vagal nerve actuation can have tonic and basal impacts that hinder the sympathetic initiation and arrival of norepinephrine at the presynaptic level. Acetylcholine discharge from parasympathetic nerve terminals will initiate ganglionic nicotinic receptors that thusly enact muscarinic receptors at the cell level. Cardiovascular impacts incorporate pulse decrease by the hindrance of the sympathetic nervous system and by direct hyperpolarization of sinus nodal cells.

Chapter 4: The Vagus Nerve And Anxiety

When we are exposed to stressful circumstances, the sympathetic nervous system is activated. If the strain continues and we can't escape what triggers it, it won't take long before issues show up. At the neurological level, this includes the involvement of two pathways: the nerve center pituitary-adrenal hub and the brain-intestine axis.

The mind reacts to stress and anxiety by expanding the production of hormones (CRFs) that transmit from the nerve center to the pituitary gland, where they initiate production of another hormone, ACTH, which thus heads out through the circulation system to the adrenal glands to stimulate cortisol and adrenaline production. These hormones function as safe framework suppressors and inflammatory precursors, which is the reason why we feel focused and we get sick effectively and, at last, we can wind up experiencing depression, a turmoil which has been connected to an inflammatory brain reaction.

Then, as though that were insufficient, constant pressure and nervousness cause an expansion in glutamate in the brain, a synapse that, when created in excess, causes a headache, depression, and anxiety. Also, an elevated level of cortisol lessens the volume of the hippocampus, the piece of the brain responsible for the formation of new memories. The contribution of the vagus nerve will lead to side effects like dizziness, gastrointestinal problems, arrhythmias, difficulty in breathing, and disproportionate emotional responses. As the vagus nerve alone can't enact the relaxation signal, the sympathetic nervous system keeps active; this will make the individual respond impulsively and suffer from anxiety.

It is curious that a study undertaken at the University of Miami found that the vagal tone is transmitted from mother to child. Women suffering from anxiety, depression, or experiencing a lot of outrage during pregnancy had lower vagal movement, and their children additionally showed low vagal action and lower levels of dopamine and serotonin.

The U.S. FDA approved VNS as a technique to prevent seizures in treatment-safe epilepsy patients in 1997, and in 2000 for treatment-resistant depression. The vagus nerve innervates the core of the single tract, which ventures to the locus coeruleus and other limbic and forebrain cortical areas. VNS builds levels of monoamines in the brain, and the locus coeruleus assumes a job in VNS-incited decrease of seizures. The current clinical act of VNS includes careful implantation of a cathode that is appended to one side cervical vagus nerve through an entry point in the neck. The anode is associated with a lead that is placed under the skin to a heartbeat generator that is subcutaneously embedded in the chest. Surgical complications, for example, disease or vocal rope impacts, happen in about 1% of patients.

Less intrusive ways to deal with invigorating the vagus nerve might be viable. In the nineteenth century, the nervous system specialist James Leonard Corning created devices to stimulate the vagus nerve transcutaneously while compacting the carotid artery, and he observed a decrease in the recurrence and length of seizures. These were not controlled examinations, and Corning abandoned the methodology due to negative reactions, for example, dizziness and syncope. Be that as it may, transcutaneous VNS (t-VNS) has recently recovered its status as a clinical treatment.

Non-invasive electrical stimulation of the vagus can be directed transcutaneously through the afferent auricular part of the nerve with electrodes clipped to the concha area of the ear. With this t-VNS, the electrical boost, with a charge that is above tactile identification yet below the pain limit, is applied through the skin to the open field of the auricular branch. Mixed results were found in an ongoing report looking at t-VNS consequences for the eradication of learned fear in people, and clinical research on the use of t-VNS is restricted, yet it is by all accounts safe and very much tolerable. Transcutaneous versions of VNS may give the advantages of VNS without the risks of medical procedure; in any case, t-VNS isn't yet a built-up treatment, and assurance of its adequacy requires further examination.

VNS holds guarantee as an assistant to presentation-based treatments since it improves memory consolidation and promotes synaptic plasticity while dampening the thoughtful pressure reaction. Although VNS has been used in humans for more than two decades, pairing it with presentation treatment has not yet been tried in patients, and numerous questions remain unanswered.

Around 80% of the cervical filaments of the left vagus nerve are tangible afferent fibers, and pre-clinical investigations are now in progress to analyze the overall commitments of PNS and CNS impacts of VNS. Individual differences in the nerve and excitement states may cause fluctuation in impacts in human patients. Recognizable proof of a solid biomarker for VNS impacts would be valuable for customizing parameters in treatment across people, and it might be used to check the potential viability of less intrusive techniques for stimulating the vagus nerve, as in t-VNS. At long last, it remains to be seen whether VNS has an intense anxiolytic impact.

According to our model, stimulation of the vagus nerve sidesteps the thoughtful reaction to risk while still promoting plasticity and the rapid consolidation of long-lasting memories. The job of the vagus nerve in the parasympathetic sensory system is to slow the thoughtful pressure reaction. Some proof shows that chronic VNS lessens nervousness in people and rats. If VNS can quickly diminish tension, this may or may not be advantageous for presentation-based treatments. It might meddle with the chance to extinguish fear from the fear response. Then again, it might rush advancements and improve consistency by cutting off the relationship between presentation to injury leads and the conditioned fear reaction during treatment. Studies are presently in progress to decide if distinctive stimulation parameters can be used to separate memory impacts of VNS from anxiolytic impacts.

During periods of development, the brain is more plastic than it is some time down the road. Quickly stored and encoded, durable memories of genuinely exciting occasions are evidence of strong neural plasticity in the adult brain.

In 1890, Harvard psychologist and philosopher William James expressed, "An experience may be so exciting emotionally as almost to leave a scar on the cerebral tissues." The neural versatility that underlies bad memories can be adaptive, reducing the probability that risky behavior will be repeated. Incidentally, traumatic memories have maladaptive outcomes, leading to nervousness and/or stress-related disorders. We plan to use the capability of the vagus nerve to drive neural plasticity during presentation treatment, while simultaneously interfering with the sympathetic fight-or-flight reaction. If effective, we will exploit components that exist to leave an enduring impact on the mind to mend the cerebral scars left by trauma.

Vagal toning is an internal, natural procedure that speaks to the function of the vagus nerve. The expansion in vagal tone initiates the parasympathetic sensory system, which means that we can loosen up more rapidly after a distressing circumstance. This will positively affect our emotional balance and health in general.

Vagus nerve incitement methods:

1. Exposure to cold. It has been noted that exposure to cold incites the vagus nerve, since it stimulates the cholinergic neurons crossing these innervations. A study conducted at the University of Oulu in Finland has revealed that ordinary exposure to cold assists with reducing the fight-or-flight response that dispatches the sympathetic nervous system.

There are additionally individuals who rest on the stomach, putting ice on the nape of the neck. Others want to drink a glass of cold water rapidly.

2. Diaphragmatic breathing. The vast majority of people breathe in air somewhere in the range of 10 and 14 times each minute, which means that they have superficial breathing. The perfect amount is to breathe in air 6 times a minute. Diaphragmatic breathing specifically initiates the vagus nerve, and the mind interprets this as being important to quiet down, regardless of whether the nerve has given that request explicitly. This system is similar to how, if you close your eyes and tap your fingers on your eyelids, you will "see" short flashes of light because the mind interprets them so.

3. Meditation, yoga, and tai-chi. Meditation can build vagal tone. This has been exhibited by scientists of Oregon University, who have seen that just five days of careful reflection promote positive emotions toward oneself. This causes vagus nerve excitation while balancing the activity of the parasympathetic sensory system, a much better outcome than conventional relaxation techniques.

Indeed, even practices like yoga and jujitsu are perfect for animating the vagus nerve.

A study at Boston University uncovered that yoga stimulates GABA neurotransmitters, which promote feelings of quiet and serenity by assisting with combatting anxiety and stress.

Vagal tone

The tone of the vagus nerve is key to actuating the parasympathetic sensory system. Vagal tone is estimated by following your heart rate and your breathing rate. Your heart rate accelerates a little when you breathe in, and slows a little when you breathe out. The greater the difference between your intake breath pulse and your exhalation heart rate, the higher your vagal tone. A higher vagal tone means that your body can loosen up quicker after experiencing stress. High vagal tone improves the capacity of many body systems, causing better glucose guidelines, diminished risk of stroke and cardiovascular illness, lower circulatory strain, improved absorption using better creation of stomach-related proteins, and decreased headaches. Higher vagal tone is additionally linked with a better temperament — not so much uneasiness, but rather more pressure flexibility.

One of the most interesting roles of the vagus nerve is that it reads the gut micro-biome and starts a reaction to balance inflammation depending on whether it identifies pathogenic versus non-pathogenic bacteria. Along these lines, the gut micro-biome can affect your temperament, feelings of anxiety, and general inflammation.

Low vagal tone is related to cardiovascular conditions and strokes, depression, diabetes, chronic fatigue syndrome, cognitive impairment, and much higher rates of inflammatory conditions. Inflammatory conditions include all autoimmune diseases, like rheumatoid joint inflammation, provocative gut infection, endometriosis, immune system thyroid conditions, lupus, and others.

How would we increase vagal tone? In the section above, we talked about increasing vagal tone using a gadget that stimulates the nerve. Fortunately, you can do this all alone, though it requires some practice. You are genetically predisposed to varying levels of vagal tone; however, this still doesn't mean that you can't work on it.

Here are a few different ways to condition the vagus nerve:

1. Slow, rhythmic, diaphragmatic breathing from your stomach, instead of shallowly from the highest point of the lungs, invigorates and conditions the vagus nerve.

2. Humming. Since the vagus nerve is associated with the vocal cords, murmuring precisely animates it. You can hum a song, or even better, repeat the sound 'OM.'

3. Talking. Talking is useful for vagal tone because of the association with the vocal cords.

4. Meditation, particularly adoring kindness meditation, increases sentiments of goodwill towards yourself as well as other people. A recent report by Barbara Fredrickson and Bethany Kik found that expanding positive feelings leads to an expanded social closeness and an improvement in vagal tone.

5. Adjusting the gut micro-biome. The nearness of solid microbes in the gut makes a positive feedback loop through the vagus nerve, expanding its tone.

The implications of such basic practices on your general wellbeing, and specifically on inflammation are broad. If you experience the ill effects of an inflammatory condition, stomach-related upset, hypertension, or depression, a more intensive take a look at vagal tone is strongly recommended. We've known for quite a long time that breathing activities and meditation are useful for our wellbeing; however, it is also interesting to gain proficiency with the mechanism by which they work. I trust this section has motivated you to start a reflective practice, as it has for me, and to search for different methods of dealing with the body's inflammatory reaction.

How it affects anxiety

Stimulating this huge nerve additionally assists with quelling anxiety. Intriguingly, yoga experts have been using the vagal reaction in breath work called pranayama as a customary piece of yoga practice for quite a long time.

According to Dr. Mladen Golubic, an internist at Cleveland Clinic's Center for Integrative Medicine, consistently practicing vagal stimulation can diminish tension and stress, and help alleviate or neutralize conditions such as asthma, incessant obstructive pulmonary disease, and cardiovascular disease. Dr. Golubic's assertion should give to every one of us a measure of comfort in that, to an enormous degree, our psychological and physical health is in our control. "There are studies that show that individuals who work on breathing activities and have those [previously mentioned] conditions – they get better," says Golubic.

Judi Bar, a yoga educator at the Cleveland Clinic, agrees with Dr. Golubic: "Our breaths will either wake us up or stimulates us. It will loosen up us, or it will balance us."

The science behind the vagal reaction

The amygdala, which is a piece of the sympathetic nervous system (SNS), gives us the flawless fight-or-flight reaction (FOF) that bothers us. Consider how you feel when some jerk cuts you off in traffic, or while waiting on hold for 20 minutes. While the FOF reaction has kept our species alive, we also get annoyed over the littlest things as a result of two almond-shaped organs at the base of our brain. People with psychological health issues, for example, chronic anxiety and depression, are continually nervous due to amygdalar activity.

When we can't relax, it's an ideal opportunity to connect with the parasympathetic nervous system (PNS) by invigorating the vagus nerve. While it might sound complicated, it's not very tough – and it turns out to be a lot simpler with standard practice. The most significant thing while stimulating the vagus nerve is to control your relaxing. Heavy breathing and a spike in pulse are side effects of the SNS FOF reaction.

"Deep breathing is an incredible case of that," says Dr. Golubic. "We have a specific space where we can control breathing. We can expand the inhalation and the exhalation. So by those practices, we can initiate the parasympathetic nervous system. The best practice is a measured breath, which includes diaphragmatic breathing."

The diaphragm is a strong, dome-shaped divider that isolates the lungs from the stomach territory. It assumes a huge job in breathing, as it is responsible for expanding the lungs. The issue is that we don't connect with the diaphragm enough while breathing; rather, we will generally breathe shallowly ("chest breathe"). When we are focused or restless, we quite often chest breathe. However, stressful times are when we need diaphragmic breathing the most.

There are significant disadvantages to not breathing with our stomach. By not drawing in with the diaphragm, our bodies don't get the ideal measure of oxygen, which therefore influences our brain and body.

Relieve anxiety instantly using this one trick

This is what you have to do:

1. Lie on your back on a level surface or a bed, with the knees marginally twisted

(you may utilize a cushion below the knees for help). Spot one hand on your upper chest and the other just below the rib cage (this will enable you to feel your stomach as you relax).

2. Breath in gradually through the nose with the goal that your stomach moves out against your hand. The hand on your chest ought to stay as still as can be.

3. Fix your stomach muscles; as you breathe out through pursed (tightly pressed) lips. The hand on your upper chest ought to stay still.

After getting acquainted with diaphragmic breathing while at the same time resting, you can do it while sitting! (Besides stages 3 and 4; there are particular differences between the two positions.) This is what to do when sitting:

1. Sit easily, with your knees twisted, and your shoulders, head, and neck loose.

2. Breathe in gradually through your nose with the goal that your stomach moves

out against your hand. The hand on the chest ought to stay stationary.

3. Spot one hand on your upper chest and the other just beneath your rib cage. (Same as in the resting position.)

4. Fix your stomach muscles; let them fix as you breathe out through pursed lips. The hand on your upper chest must stay still.

Per the Cleveland Clinic, practice these activities for 5 to 10 minutes, at least 3 times every day. Gradually increase the time, as you feel suitable. You can also ease yourself into it by just putting your face in super cold water.

Singing, humming, chanting, and gargling

The vagus nerve is associated with your vocal cords and the muscles at the rear of your throat. Singing, humming, chanting, and gargling can engage these muscles and stimulate your vagus nerve.

3. Acupuncture

Acupuncture is another elective treatment that has been appeared to stimulate the vagus nerve. I'm a huge fan of auricular acupuncture. Auricular acupuncture is the practice of having needles embedded in the ear. I'd advise attempting to discover a wellbeing expert in your vicinity who gives it, particularly if you're weaning off medications. It truly helped me the first time I fell off antidepressants. I was shocked.

Research shows that ear needle therapy stimulates the vagus nerve, increases vagal action and vagal tone, and can help treat neurodegenerative diseases using the vagal guideline. **4. Yoga and Tai Chi**

Yoga and tai chi are two "personality body" relaxation methods that work by stimulating the vagus nerve and expanding the action of your parasympathetic "rest and relaxation" nervous system. Studies have demonstrated that yoga produces GABA, a calming synapse in your mind. Scientists believe that it does this by stimulating vagal afferents, which increase movement in the parasympathetic nervous system. Researchers have also found that yoga invigorates the vagus nerve and accordingly ought to be practiced by individuals who battle depression and/or anxiety.

Judo has additionally been shown to build heart rate variability, and specialists figure this implies it can enhance vagal modulation.

6. Probiotics

It's getting progressively more obvious to specialists that gut microorganisms improve brain function by influencing the vagus nerve. In one study, animals were given the probiotic Lactobacillus rhamnosus, and scientists discovered positive changes to the GABA receptors in their brain, a decrease in pressure hormones, and less depression and anxiety-like behavior. The researchers also presumed that these useful changes between the gut and the mind were encouraged by the vagus nerve. When the vagus nerve was removed in other mice, the expansion of Lactobacillus rhamnosus to their stomach-related frameworks neglected to reduce anxiety, stress, or improve mood.

I recently explored some different ways you can nourish the awesome microorganisms in your gut.

7. Meditation and neurofeedback

Meditation is my preferred relaxation strategy, and it can animate the vagus nerve and increase vagal tone. Research shows that reflection increases vagal tone and positive feelings, and promotes feelings of goodwill toward yourself. Another examination found that contemplation decreases sympathetic fight or flight action and increases vagal regulation. Reciting "om," which is frequently done during meditation, has additionally been appeared to animate the vagus nerve.

I was unable to discover any research substantiating this; however, as far as I can tell, neurofeedback increased my pulse fluctuation and vagal tone as estimated by my EmWave2. Since I've done neurofeedback, I use the Muse headband to meditate. Like neurofeedback, it gives you continuous input on your brainwaves.

8. Omega-3 fatty acids

Omega-3 unsaturated fats are basic fats that your body can't create itself. They are found primarily in fish and are essential for the ordinary electrical workings of your brain and nervous system. In any case, scientists have additionally found that omega-3 unsaturated fats increase vagal tone and vagal activity. Studies have demonstrated that they reduce heart rate and increase heart rate variability, which means they likewise stimulate the vagus nerve. And, high fish intake is likewise connected with "upgraded vagal action and parasympathetic predominance." This is the reason I eat heaps of wild-caught salmon, and take a supplement of krill oil.

9. Exercise

Exercise increases your brain's growth hormone, supports your brain's mitochondria, and helps reverse cognitive decline. At the same time, it's been shown to stimulate the vagus nerve, which may clarify its physical and mental health impacts. Many mental health specialists prescribe exercise as their main suggestion for improved brain health.

This is my activity schedule:

Lift heavy weights 1-4 times per week

High-intensity interval sprinting 1-2 times per week

Walk as much as I can (ideally 30-60 minutes every day)

Walking, weightlifting, and sprinting are the best types of activity, but you should pick a game or exercise schedule that you like, so you'll stay with it reliably.

10. Zinc

As I've talked about previously, zinc is a basic mineral for psychological health, particularly if you battle with chronic anxiety. One study showed that zinc assists with vagus nerve stimulation in zinc-deficient rats. It's estimated that 2 billion individuals on the planet are deficient in zinc, and six distinct studies show that subclinical insufficiency of zinc restricts brain function in youngsters and adults. In this way, if you battle with a brain or emotional health issue, it's very possible that you're zinc-deficient. Probably the best food sources of zinc include clams, grass-fed meat, pumpkin seeds, cashews, mushrooms, and spinach. However, I still recommend supplementation to guarantee you get enough. I made and took the Optimal Zinc supplement to ensure my zinc levels are ideal. Look at my last post about zinc and copper in case you're keen on finding more supplements you can take to increase your zinc levels.

11. Massage

Research shows that massage can invigorate the vagus nerve, and increase vagal movement and vagal tone. The vagus nerve can also be stimulated by massaging a few specific areas of the body. Foot massages (reflexology) have appeared to boost vagal modulation and heart rate variability, and decrease the fight or flight sympathetic reaction. Rubbing the carotid sinus, a zone situated close to the right side of your throat, can also stimulate the vagus nerve to lessen seizures. I, for one, get a back rub from a certified specialist every couple of months.

12. Socializing and laughing

I've just examined how socializing and laughing can decrease your body's principal stress hormone. Also, presently I've discovered that they likely do this by stimulating the vagus nerve. Scientists have found that reflecting on positive social interactions improves vagal tone and increases positive feelings. Chuckling has been shown to increase heart-rate variability and improve state of mind. The reverse is also true: vagus nerve stimulation regularly prompts chuckling as a symptom, suggesting that they are associated and impact each other. Therefore, my recommendation is to hang out and chuckle with your friends as much as could reasonably be expected.

13. Intermittent fasting

On most days, I don't have any breakfast, and I break my fast" by eating my first meal of the day around 2 or 3 p.m. That means I eat all my nourishment for the day within an 8-hour window. There are numerous medical advantages to doing this. As I've talked about previously, intermittent fasting can support your brain's development hormone, improve mitochondrial work, and may assist some people in overcoming brain fog and cognitive decline. Research also shows that fasting and caloric limitation increases heart rate variability, which is an indicator that it increases parasympathetic action and vagal tone.

The ideal approach to begin fasting is basically by having supper around 6, not eating anything after that before bed, and having a standard breakfast the following day. That should give you around 12-14 hours of fasting time.

Chapter 5: Why Vagal Tone Matters

The vagal tone is how good and "sound" the nerve of the Vagus is. The higher the vagal tone, the easier it is to get into a state of relaxation.

Research published in 2013 in Psychological Science reveals a positive feedback loop between high vagal tone, good physical health, and good emotional health. While the researchers agree that "the processes underlying the relationship between positive emotions and physical health remain a mystery," they identified a link between a toned Vagal nerve and better physical and emotional health. The reverse is true, as well. The better the physical and emotional health, the higher the sound of your Vagal.

What Does The Body's Vagus Nerve Do?

In optimal health, the vagus nerve is an important player, particularly when entering a parasympathetic or comfortable state. Here are some of the reasons the body is affected by the Vagus nerve.

Connects The Brain To The Gut

If you've ever had a gut sensation about something, it's due to your vagus nerve. The vagus nerve links the brain to the intestine and sends information back and forth. This is also called the axis of the intestinal brain. Your gut tells details about your brain by electrical impulses called "potentials of action."

Connects The Brain To Other Organs

The vagus nerve also connects the brain with other vital organs as it passes to the intestine. This takes sensory information to the brain from the liver.

When regulating the heart rate, the vagus nerve plays an important role. The neurotransmitter acetylcholine is activated by the vagus nerve, which decreases the heart rate. The improvement in cardiac levels includes vagus nerve stimulation suppression (which ensures no release of acetylcholine). Physicians will monitor your heart rate variability (HRV) and figure out a lot about your heart and vagus nerve's wellbeing. If your HRV is low, there's a high vagal tone.

The vagus nerve also plays a role in the operation of the heart. Often responsible for telling the lungs to breathe is the acetylcholine that the vagus nerve induces to release.

Controls The Parasympathetic Nervous System

The parasympathetic nervous system is the nervous system's "stop and eats" component (as opposed to the sympathetic nervous system's fight or flight mechanism). As described above, the vagus nerve activates the release of acetylcholine (in relaxation) to suppress heart rate. The vagus nerve also plays an important role in calming and regeneration stimulation.

Stimulates Digestive Tract

It is the vagus nerve, which activates digestion. Even before eating any food, it does this. To start producing gastric juices to prepare for digestion, it sends signals to the gastrointestinal (GI) tract. If the vagus nerve is not optimal, it is not optimal for digestion.

Stimulates Memory Making

Research by the University of Virginia showed that activation of the vagus nerve could help to solidify memories by inducing norepinephrine release. In those with memory problems or those with Alzheimer's disease, this can be significant.

Prevents Chronic Inflammation

One of the vagus nerve's most remarkable features is that it can stop inflammation. In many modern diseases, from cancer to heart disease, chronic inflammation is involved. According to a Molecular Medicine study, when the vagus nerve detects inflammation (for instance, by the existence of pro-inflammatory cytokine), it activates the production of anti-inflammatory neurotransmitters to control the immune system.

However, a 2016 study found that activation of the vagus nerve helped to reduce signs of rheumatoid arthritis, a condition without a cure.

Natural Ways ToStimulate The Vagus Nerve

Stimulation of the vagus nerve is necessary for optimum health. There is a system approved by the FDA that can be inserted in the skin. To activate the vagus nerve, it emits electrical impulses. However, without surgery, appliances, or side effects, there are other ways to activate the vagus nerve.

Cold Therapy

Cold therapy has many benefits from faster recovery from exercise and improved immune function. Acute cold exposure, according to a 2001 report, also stimulates the vagus nerve and cholinergic neurons and nitrergic neurons through vagus nerve pathways. This means that cold exposure can also increase parasympathetic function through the nerve of the vagus, suppressing the sympathetic response (fighting and flight).

Deep Breathing

Deep, slow breathing can help induce relaxation; it is well-known. Vagal stimulation, as mentioned earlier, can cause relaxation, but the opposite is true as well. Relaxation may stimulate the nerve of the vagus. So inducing deep breathing, relaxation can help improve vagal tone. In the future, this will make it easier to enter a relaxed state!

Singing, Humming, Gargling

Singing or humming on their own may be soothing, but there is a physiological reason for it. The vocal cords are attached to the vagus nerve. Research published in Psychology's Frontiers reveals that it can be triggered by chanting, humming, and even gargling. Chewing also increases the operation of the vagus nerve (and the parasympathetic process, which controls digestion, making sense!). While it may have its downsides, it means chewing gum often activates the vagus nerve.

Intermittent Fasting

Intermittent fasting can enhance mental and mitochondrial function. It can also improve metabolism and reduce heart disease and cancer risk.

But it turns out that these health benefits can be correlated with the ability of intermittent fasting to activate the vagus nerve and enhance the vagal tone. A 2003 study found fasting to be a vagus nerve biochemical activator.

Wave Vibration

The scientific community has studied wave vibration heavily for its health benefits. This treatment involves sitting on a low-level vibration oscillating surface. Then these vibrations create positive stress throughout the body (like the type of stress that exercise creates). This stress, among other parts of the body, activates the vagal nerve.

Probiotics

Probiotics are an important part of the diet and benefit from digestive problems and skin problems for many illnesses. Probiotics can also be useful in stimulating the vagus nerve, and it turns out. Results from a 2011 study found that giving Lactobacillus Rhamnosus mice increased their development of GABA and decreased stress, as well as activity related to depression and anxiety.

Ironically, those who had not had a vagus nerve in the probiotics (it was removed) did not see the same effects. This suggests that there was something to do with the activation of the vagus nerve to improve stress resilience.

Healthy Fats AndOmega-3s

A study published in Frontiers in Psychology in 2011 found that high fish intake was associated with a primary parasympathetic (relaxed) nervous system and decreased vagal activity. Scientists speculated that the explanation for this was the fish's omega-3 quality.

Exercise

In a healthy lifestyle, exercising is an important part. But it seems that stimulating the vagus nerve may also be beneficial. This may be the explanation of why we can cope with exercise. One study in 2010 found that mild exercise stimulated gastric emptying and enhanced digestion. They figured out this was due to vagal stimulation.

Massage

Research suggests that in relaxing the vagus nerve, acupuncture can be helpful. There was a greater weight gain attributed to vagal operation in one 2012 study of premature infants who were massaged. We're trying to use a range of massage techniques and tools at home; this is one factor.

Foot reflexology can also improve the sound of the vagus. Foot reflexology improved vagal stimulation, reduced sympathetic regulation, and lowered blood pressure, according to a study published in Alternative Therapies in Health and Medicine.

Laughter and Social Enjoyment

We all know that a good way to relax is to smile and be around friends and family. But a report in 2013 stumbled upon an interesting finding: there is a connection between mental health and social enjoyment of physical health. Positive social experiences affect positive emotions, which enhance the sound of the vagus. It enhanced physical health afterward.

The study concluded that in a self-sustaining upward-spiral environment, "positive emotions, positive social interactions, and physical health impact each other." The study also found that regular meditation and constructive reinforcement can bring people into this upward spiral.

Acupuncture

The use of acupuncture by ancient Chinese medicine may be useful to activate the vagus nerve. Research shows that ear acupuncture can benefit from the following:

☐ Heart regulation

☐ Respiratory regulation

☐ Gastrointestinal tract regulation

Additionally, according to a 2012 report, foot reflexology can reduce blood pressure by modulating the vagus nerve.

Chapter 6: The Safekeeping Of The Vagus Nerve

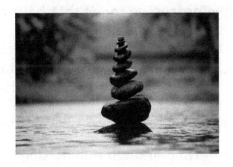

Brain Balance

First, you have to make sure your brain is balanced. Without a balanced nervous system, your efforts to eliminate chronic pain will be wasted. Many things can cause brain imbalances. Most common are head injuries and exposure to electromagnetic radiation from personal wireless devices.

Things that increase brain imbalance risk factors include:

- Using Bluetooth devices and cell phones, walkie talkies, using desktop and laptop computers and iPads.

- Eating processed foods that have MSG.

- Consuming drinks containing artificial sweeteners, and drinking fluoridated water.

- Leading a stressful life.

- Not getting enough quality sleep.

Brain Balancing Using Affirmations

Studies show that when the thymus gland is balanced, both hemispheres of the brain also remain balanced and serve to lower chronic pain. The nice thing about affirmations is that they don't cost you anything; you just have to repeat the affirmations regularly throughout the day to keep your brain in balance. You need to "feel" the words to get full benefits.

The following is a list of daily affirmations:

- I have faith, gratitude, trust, love and courage.

- I'm modest, I'm humble and tolerant.

- I'm clean and good, I deserve to be loved.

- I'm content and tranquil.

- I have forgiveness in my heart.

- My life energy is high, life is full of love.

Brain Balancing Music

Brain balancing music encourages a balanced nervous system and balances both hemispheres of the brain. Brain balancing music uses three coordinated methods: "primordial sounds", "brainwave entrainment", and "multi-layered music" to bring the mind-body into a deeply relaxed and balanced state. You have to listen to the music on a daily basis to maintain your brain balance which is crucial for health and healing of chronic pain.

Avoid GMO foods

GMO or genetically modified organisms have been introduced to our diets over the past decade. As of this writing, the GMO foods are not labeled in the U. S. So, the average American's is unconsciously consuming GMO rich canola oil, sugar. beets, corn, soy and cottonseed oil. GMO foods can cause all sorts of gastrointestinal problems, allergies, weight gain, and immune problems. Avoiding GMO foods can reduce or even eliminate many health problems, including chronic pain.

Emotional Freedom Techniques

This amazing technique deals swiftly with all sorts of emotional pain and has an infinite number of applications. EFT has been around for quite a while and is now used in many hospitals and psych units throughout the world by professional psychologists and psychiatrists who are continuing to get very positive results with severe emotional pain and trauma.

There is no doubt that strong emotions can be very painful things and it is now recognized that emotion follows thought. This is why psychiatrists spend years talking about trauma and trying to uncover triggers and thoughts that cause bad feelings, depression, phobias and the like.

EFT is a great way to deal with all fear though you will have to be thorough. Really take a look at all the different aspects of that fear and treat each one with a very specific opening statement.

Emotional Freedom Technique (EFT) or tapping requires that you tap specific acupressure points on the torso, hands and on the head in order to clear energy blocks caused by negative emotions and feelings.

What you do is tap lightly on each of them. You get used to doing this very quickly, and when you have been using EFT for a while you can just do a few taps here and there, maybe on your collarbone or under your eye, for rapid relief.

Generally tapping involves two stages. In the first stage you are tapping to express the negative emotions. This stage of tapping will last as long as you have an emotional charge, continual tapping will bring that charge down to a minimal level.

The second stage includes reframing the condition positively where you choose a positive emotion or thought to replace the negative ones. The cool thing is you can't tap incorrectly; your intention is enough to make it work correctly. Even without tapping the right acupressure points, you will still release the negative energy from your body.

Basic EFT instructions

Choose a negative emotion or feeling you wish to clear based on a situation that is troubling you. For example, you might be angry at your neighbor Tom for letting his dog poop in your backyard.

First, feel where in your body the negative emotions are contained and tap there. This may be one location or many. When you feel your emotional charge has dropped significantly and want to move on to the positive rounds, then tap all the acupressure points again and review your state of feelings. For example, as you tap, you might say, "I choose to be open", "I choose forgiveness", "I choose to let go and move on",etc.

Cultivating a Positive Attitude

The easiest way I know to create a positive attitude is to count your blessings. I know, I know, that may sound like old hat, something you've tried a hundred times, you think there's nothing to be thankful for, but look closely and start really small.

First of all, concentrate on small things then you will find them extending out, past the current moment. Remember, start small, if you have beautiful strong nails, list those, if you like the way your old slippers keep your feet snuggly warm, list those. Become aware of the tiniest pleasures throughout the day and mentally add them to your list.

Now do that three times a day. It only takes moments. You can write them down if you wish. First thing in the morning, lunchtime and before bed. Make it a rule and do it for at least a week.

So, the goal is to create an attitude of gratefulness, for what you DO have, and in this way, you open the floodgates for a whole lot more of the same. Whatever your beliefs on the subject it is an inescapable fact that like attracts like, whether that is misery or joy, so you may as well choose joy!

Visualization and Setting Goals

Visualization and setting goals are important. You should have one big goal – to fully heal and return to normal, or an even better life – and some small milestones you will set for yourself.

Visualizing a life where you are painless and is free to do whatever you want can help in cementing your determination to heal. This will also keep you up when the emotionally-taxing treatment brings you a bit down. By setting a final goal at the end of smaller goals, the big one feels easier. This is achieved by slowly traversing through the smaller goals one by one. Set a daily or weekly goal and visualize what you will be able to think and do by the end of that time period. Always give yourself some time to feel the celebration of your accomplishment for every milestone. Not only will it give you a needed break in your climb towards betterment, you will also feel more encouraged to go on and reach the final goal.

Guided imagery, or creative visualization as it is commonly called, is another alternative therapy that can be used in pain management. This method involves focusing the imagination on certain positive events or behaviors that you would like to occur in the future. The principle behind this practice is that the mind and the body are connected and they influence each other. The emotional trauma associated with some physical injuries and events can be replaced by these self-suggestions, positive images, and creative imaginary techniques.

Many researchers have stated that visualization is one of the most effective and powerful tools of change. It can have a great positive impact on the patient if guided correctly. Visualization can be done independently or under another's guidance. But most researchers opine that it is more effective when somebody else guides you through the process as you respond more quickly to the guidance of an external voice.

There are numerous ways to start the process of visualization. If you are practicing it independently, there are many CD's available online and in retail outlets that can guide you through the process.

Utilizing visualization for pain management is a powerful technique. By doing this, the brain starts to respond to the inputs given in the form of two-dimensional images. Then the brain sends out the signal for the body to relax. Therefore, by imagining the situation where you don't feel any pain, the body relaxes as the brain starts responding to those stimuli. This technique is very effective in treating different types of health issues both physical and emotional.

Visualization should ideally be performed in a quiet area where you will not be disturbed or distracted. It is best to keep the lighting dim or even maintain total darkness. Each of the sessions may last from 20 minutes to an hour and you may start feeling slight positive changes from the very first session.

Music Therapy

Music therapy offers numerous health benefits, but it is frequently used for physical and mental pain management. It helps to relieve stress and anxiety, which is often exasperated by pain, as well as giving you a mood boost when you are experiencing chronic pain.

It should create a gentle and relaxing response in the person listening to the music, which if done right, can help them reduce their pain or at least help them handle it better.

With just a little research, you can experiment with music therapy on your own, or seek out a licensed musical therapist who has gone through a training program.

Your music therapy program might include listening to music or getting you involved in making music, writing songs, or just singing along to songs.

There are several reasons to give it a try.

- You may not need to use as much pain medication, which can cause other body issues, can become addictive, and eventually stop working.

- If you find it is helping, add it to your antipain arsenal, as it is a good, ongoing therapy that can help with long-term pain management.

- The fact that it can reduce stress and help your body relax, is often why it often works for chronic pain management.

- This will help improve your overall quality of life naturally.

- Find a professional to learn more about music therapy if you would like to explore this natural method for helping with your chronic pain.

Comfort yourself

Comfort and give advice to yourself as if you're helping your best friend, or a close family member. You are your greatest friend and your closest family after all; just as you are your worst enemy. It works both ways, you know. Of course, such an activity that requires clarity of thought and focus of your mind requires that you, yourself have identified what exactly is wrong. So, dig in and help that pain-filled, trembling you inside that is experiencing a darkened interior of your heart.

Letting Go

It is very painful to blame yourself for something that you have no control over. Guilt and self-judgment is one of the leading causes for chronic pain symptoms and are usually either self-imposed or are drilled into someone throughout a significant period of time. It could also be an experience long gone in the past that no one can do anything about anymore. In such cases, letting go would be the best option. One cannot totally forget memories, especially those that are heavy enough to cause impacts that affect you physically in the present. But they can be accepted, acknowledged and regarded as valuable stepping stones for the current you to reach where you are now. Don't endanger the future for something that happened in the past. Let them be your inspiration, your motivation to keep moving forward and up, instead of taking them with you like shackles that remind you of the pain. Don't live in the past, gradually move on into the present and be hopeful for your future.

Biofeedback

Biofeedback is a special technique that helps people to improve their health by training them to control certain involuntary processes of the body. Using the biofeedback mechanism, the individual learns to change his physiological activity in order to improve health conditions and performance levels.

You may think biofeedback is not a self-help technique to eliminate chronic pain, but it is really an effective method. Biofeedback is helpful for everything from gastric distress, high blood pressure, migraine headaches, anxiety, sleep disorders and muscle pains. Biofeedback is generally done under supervision of a health professional, but with a little training you can do it yourself. Basically, biofeedback involves listening to a relaxation tape and having a small electrode taped to one of your fingers.

Biofeedback sessions can take 15 to 30 minutes and during that time you will be using guided imagery and relaxation breathing. While you are practicing relaxing methods, you can see your heart rate or skin temperature in the monitor.

The therapy involves attaching electrodes to the skin, which displays the results to a connected monitor and this is the information that is used to help control your involuntary functions. There is no exact evidence on how the biofeedback technique works, but many experiments conducted by researchers have reported that it gives relief from stress and helps the body to relax, which is vital for maintaining good health.

Relaxation Training

Relaxation training involves employing some innovative methods of stress and pain management. The techniques are geared at helping you keep up with your day to day activities with ease. Relaxation is not just enjoying a good movie or watching a game, relaxation happens when both mind and body are calm, de-stressed and in-sync with each other. The best part about relaxation training is that it is free of cost, takes relatively little time and it can be practiced anywhere. Whether you are travelling or sitting in the office, you can spare a few minutes to unwind. The goal of this relaxation therapy, like any other alternative therapy, is to avoid the use of traditional medicine and treat the problem as naturally as possible.

Meditation and Mindfulness

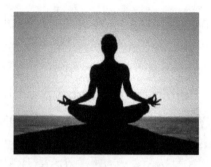

It is human nature to worry, but when those worries consume and inhibit you and your daily life, then you know it's time to take control of your mind. Meditation is a highly effective tool to recenter your head and control your thought patterns. When you are trapped in your head with anxious thoughts, your brain is conditioned to think negatively. Your automatic reaction is to think of every worst-case scenario. This is a vicious cycle, and one that may seem impossible to break. Don't be discouraged, you have the power to demolish your inhibitions and take back your mind.

Meditation allows you ample time with yourself away from listening to what everyone is telling you about your condition. Every time you are anxious, take a deep breath and maintain a steady relationship with your breathing and take notice of your surroundings, the natural sounds around you and your body's response to the stimuli being introduced to your senses.

Meditation is a practice wherein a person induces an alternate level consciousness or trains his mind to practice stillness. There are a variety of techniques for promoting relaxation, establishing stillness, and building internal energy. When you meditate, you relax your mind and body. Meditation should be done in a quiet and peaceful place in order to attain peace of mind. You can do meditation alone or in a group.

Meditation can offer profound rest to your physiological self by activating a parasympathetic response in the nervous system, also known as the relaxation response. Essentially, rest is a natural way of getting rid of anxiety and stress. Your body is designed to eliminate stress when you sleep.

Today, there are a lot of stressors around. You can get stressed out from your daily activities, the people around you, and the situations that you are in. If you want to have a healthier mind and body, meditation may be the relief you have been looking for.

Simply put, meditation is the practice of awareness. It is awareness of your thoughts, your body, and who you are. Meditation involves ridding your mind of the abundant chaos in the outside world, and focusing on the condition of your own spirit. It is easy to get caught up in what is happening externally, and meditation teaches you who you are aside from your racing thoughts. There are different ways to practice meditation, all of which focus on different types of mindfulness. All of them are beneficial in overcoming anxiety.

Meditation is broadly known to help with pain management and relief. Unlike the methods already mentioned, meditation brings relaxation, clarity, and healing to the whole self without any particular focus on specific components or issues. Meditation makes minds, intuitions, and bodies operate more efficiently. Combining this with whatever level or kind of yoga you can tolerate will enhance the benefits of each.

Meditation can be described as a state of deep peace that occurs as a result of a calm and stress-free mind. What you will discover, however, is that the peace and serenity that you find during your meditation sessions, carries over into other areas of your life when you are not actively involved in meditation.

It has been proven that stress and anxiety are at the root of many health issues. When you integrate meditation into your life, it will lower your stress and anxiety levels, boost your morale and reduce the pain symptoms associated with psychosomatic conditions.

Chapter 7: An Introduction To The Polyvagal Theory

Developmental outcomes, physiology, and social engagement are explored in the neurobiological theory, the polyvagal theory. It is a complicated theory that can get convoluted. The design of this chapter is to help break down the theory into a three-part introduction. To begin, you need to know more about stress and the physiology of it as well as various responses to stress that occur in your body.

Your Nervous System

There are two primary nervous systems in your body, your peripheral nervous system, or PNS, and your central nervous system, or CNS. The CNS is your spinal cord and brain. It controls thoughts. The PNS is all the other nerves as well as ganglia. These regulate the limbs, organs, and muscles. In the PNS is the autonomic nervous system, or ANS, and the somatic nervous system. Both are responsible for involuntary and voluntary functioning. For example, talking, seeing, smelling, as well as digesting and breathing. Then the ANS is broken down to the parasympathetic and sympathetic nervous system. This is the "fight, flight, or freeze" impulse and "rest and digest." When you relax and let yourself be calm, you signal your parasympathetic nervous system to "rest and digest." But if you become afraid or stressed, you have a physiological response. This is your sympathetic nervous system, or your "fight, flight, or freeze" response. Your body is responding to mobilize and handle the "threat." Your heart beats faster, pupils dilate, saliva production increases, and your blood sugar increases.

When you are threatened or afraid, the model is fairly straightforward. Your body responds to a problem. But there are a lot of things that are still unanswered or are a variable. For instance, is there always either a parasympathetic response or a sympathetic response or can you operate without one of those responses? How does the body respond when the body is chronically stressed? Why does a body trigger the "fight, flight, or freeze" response when you see something dramatic on television when you know it is not real or is not life-threatening. Are emotions necessary for these responses?

Humans are "hard-wired" to be social and in groups. This means that social engagement is entangled with how you respond physiologically. This has led to humans coping with stressors that are urgent and impactful on the immediate self but also stressors that are social in nature, too. This theory, the polyvagal theory, attempts to stitch together factors of these such responses on a social, physiological, and evolutionary platform. But before getting into these factors, it is good to have a review of the Vagus nerve and how it deals with the regulation of your stress levels.

The Vagus Nerve and Stress Regulation

This "wandering" nerve that stretches from your brainstem to your colon has about 80% of its nerve fibers working in one capacity; to send information from the organs in your body to your brain. This type of nerve fiber is called afferent fibers. This information alerts your brain about what your organs are doing, like if your heart is beating at a normal rate or faster, or if you are having trouble with digestion or if it is functioning properly, or if your pupils are dilated or not. The other almost 20% of the nerves are efferent, or "highways" for the brain to tell your organs to do different things. This will be discussed in more detail later in this chapter. The Vagus nerve has a very important role in the regulation of the body. Its primary job is to make sure everything is balanced with one another.

This is called "homeostasis." This relates to things like body temperature, chemistry in your body, activation, etc. And what is even more amazing is that the homeostasis of an organ can be different depending on the context of the situation, meaning the Vagus nerve interprets the context in which you are living and works with the organs to respond evenly to that.

To help illustrate this point, think about what happens to your body when the weather is hot. Blood takes a longer route, moving around your body to spread out the heat, but when the temperatures drop and it is cold outside, your blood changes its average course, favoring your major organs over your extremities. Even the arteries in your legs and arms constrict in the cold to minimize the amount of blood flowing into them so it can keep your organs warm. It may be frustrating to suffer from cold fingers and toes but it is your body's way of keeping your body temperature balanced for your internal organs. Next time you experience this, take a moment to thank your Vagus nerve for doing its job and put on warmer clothing without complaint!

Social stressors can also change the equilibrium of your body. The average heart beats between 60 and 80 times every minute when it is relaxed. But if a bear chases you, or you are running a marathon, your heart should pump faster to spread more oxygen out. In both scenarios, the primary goal for your body is to go a further distance. The extra blood and oxygen are being utilized to help you reach that goal. But when you feel nervous or see something disturbing on television your heart also picks up the pace. Think about before the first day of work, the morning of a big exam, preparing to walk on stage for a large presentation, etc. All of these situations typically lead to a faster heart rate. These situations may seem strange to have more blood and oxygen racing around your body. You are not preparing your body to fight or run, but your body is responding like it is. It is acting the same as if a bear all of a sudden rounded the corner to maul you, instead of just saying hello to a nice, attractive, special person. These "other" situations are explained in the polyvagal theory to define why this happens.

"Polyvagal" is used to describe the branches of the Vagus nerve. There are two types; unmyelinated and myelinated. A Myelin Sheath is a substance primarily made of fat that lines various nerves. It is meant to aid signals so they are sent to the brain faster and more accurately. If a nerve does not have a myelin sheath, it is called unmyelinated and it functions more primitively. The messaging from these nerves is not as fast or organized. To help you visualize the difference between the two, think about cars traveling on a well-designed and maintained road with strategic stoplights and a speed limit sign. The road is designed to help passengers travel quickly and easily but is controlled to maintain the safety of all the passengers on it. This is a "myelinated" road. Now visualize a dirt road winding around backcountry with no regulations in place and no clear direction. The journey is more troublesome and dangerous for all the travels passing along it. In addition, with the bumps and the uneven surface, it is harder to travel quickly. This is an "unmyelinated" road.

The branches of the Vagus nerve, and all the nerves in the body, are meant to keep your body balanced and functioning well. This is accomplished with three neural control stages. These three stages are operating in the unmyelinated branch of the Vagus nerve, the sympathetic adrenal system, and the myelinated branch of the Vagus nerve. There are different times for operation and a variety of effects each stage produces in and on the body when it is activated.

The unmyelinated branch of the Vagus nerve can be considered the least evolved of all the stages. This is because it is a more primitive evolution of communication in the body, and it is seen in primitive vertebrates, amphibians, and various reptiles as well. As animals evolved, coping skills for stress evolved to be more effective on a physiological level.

Below is a table that outlines the different stages, from least evolved to the most, along with the behavioral functions each stage deals with.

Stage Number	Component Utilized	Behavior and Function	"Lower Motor Neurons"
3	Myelinated branch of the Vagus nerve	Inhibits sympathetic -adrenal influences,	Nucleus ambiguus

		related to calming and social-soothing as well as social communication	
2	Sympathetic-adrenal System	Actively avoiding, mobilization	Spinal cord
1	Unmyelinated branch of the Vagus nerve	Passive avoidance, feigning death, immobilized	Dorsal motor nucleus of the Vagus nerve

There is a fine balance struck between inhibition and excitation. This means that when one is active, the others are inactive. When one is "on," the others are "off."

When you are facing common, everyday stress, like a deadline at work of having a fight with your partner or having a lot of homework to do, your body tends to suppress two states, favoring the reliance on your more evolved step, the myelinated Vagus nerve. But when stress becomes too great, your body drops to the next stage, which is more primitive. And then further, if compounded.

Unmyelinated Vagus Nerve Introduction

This is the most primitive response to your environment. This is about immobilization or even fainting, which is common in humans at this stage. Animals feign death when activating their unmyelinated Vagus nerve. The main goal of this response is to conserve your resources. This is especially seen in your heart rate. Bradycardia, or a low, maintained heart rate, is often the outcome of this state. Some animals and most reptiles use this to mimic death, but humans need more oxygen than these animals. In fact, all mammals would suffer severe damage if they feigned death in this manner. To see examples of this, research sharks when they go into the "shark trance" or snakes when they experience tonic immobility. It is clear that this response is not always very effective, which is most likely why humans have evolved to not use this response often. You probably will not be in this stage on a regular basis, certainly not during your day-to-day activities. This stage is activated only when there is extreme stress.

If someone experiences this stress and response chronically, they suffer from an illness called "vasovagal syncope." These people faint when they are triggered in different situations or experience extreme stress. Emotional triggers are also known to cause this response for people with this diagnosis, such as seeing blood. It can also occur from standing too long. It is unknown what causes this disorder but some experiments conducted on animals suggest it is the sudden activation of the unmyelinated Vagus nerve that creates this result. In addition, this disorder can be a life-long struggle or it can appear only when a person is under extreme stress.

Sympathetic – Adrenal System

This second stage in the profess mobilizes the "fight, flight or freeze" response. When your body detects a threat, it can respond in this primitive fashion. This response uses up a lot of energy and therefore typically only engage it when there is a threat to your environment that makes you feel unsafe. The activation of this response is often subconscious because we are constantly observing and analyzing the environment. This is called neuroception. You may not know it, but you are constantly evaluating the places and situations you are in to determine if you are safe or threatened.

There is a difference between neuroception, perception, and sensation.

The sensation is how your body receives an input from the senses and is a completely physiological response. Perception, on the other hand, is how you process the various sensations you experience. People can sense the same things, like look at the same picture, but they perceive it differently. Neuroception does not align with either of these experiences. It is all about how you decide if something is safe or not for you. For instance, you may not think the disagreement you are having with someone is unsafe or threatening, but your mind interprets clues like facial expressions, tone of voice, appearance, and decide it is a threat to you. This is a subconscious interpretation of stimuli and cues appearing in that context. You are not just perceiving the stimuli but also deciding if the environment you are in is safe or not because of that stimuli. This is a great response to have evolved because it allows animals and humans to leave once a predator is perceived.

This is a response best for physical danger, but sometimes it is activated in psychologically stressing situations, as well. For instance, you want to speak to a special person you want to make a good impression on. During an encounter with this person, something happens where you become embarrassed. On the outside, you may appear calm, or you may try to tell yourself to calm down, but often your face will reveal what is happening. Your face may turn red and become hot. Your heartbeat increases. Palms become sweaty. These responses are part of the sympathetic-adrenal system. There is an emotional threat present that your body perceived and it is responding as if that were a physical threat to your life. For animals, this is very helpful. But for humans in day-to-day societal and social engagement, it is not the most adaptive response stage.

The third stage in the process is the most complex. It is integrated and evolved to allow you to interact with your environment in a high-functioning manner. This is called the "social engagement system." This system regulates face and head striated muscles and the visceral organs regulated by the myelinated Vagus nerve. It is a two-part process; it first regulates the psychological "distance" from threats, and then by straining engagement and stimuli from other situations. As an example, when infants recognize the face of their mothers, they feel a sense of security. The process reduces the "distance" between the infant and the mother by listening to her voice and using their vocal abilities to communicate with her. To increase the engagement the infant may then make sure to keep their eyes open and trained on their mother, as well as shift their body to face her more. This system is responsible for controlling facial muscles, meaning it is valuable in communicating emotions and showing listening skills and visual recognition. All the individual functions involved use a large number of cranial nerves thanks to the neural circuit system. All of this starts in the cortex.

When you feel threatened, your stage 2, "fight, flight, or freeze," sympathetic-adrenal system is triggered. When you are secure and safe, your stage 3, "social engagement system," myelinated Vagus nerve is triggered. This stage 3 inhibits the response to stress and activates the nerves in the cranium to encourage engagement. In this process, the Vagus nerve is just one of the cranial nerves stimulated.

Throughout this process, it is important to recognize that animals primarily only had an unmyelinated Vagus nerve to activate the parasympathetic action. Over time mammals evolved to have the myelinated Vagus nerve as well to align social engagement with parasympathetic action.

In the medulla, the various cranial nerves converge with the Vagus nerve. Here, they can instigate responses that are similar and coordinated. For instance, when there is a feeling of security, the medulla in the brainstem signals various cranial nerves to align activity and social engagement. This requires the Vagus nerve to be an active participant in the social engagement system in your body.

The Vagal Tone

There are a lot of cranial nerves engaging in the system, with many parallel functions as the Vagus nerve, so it stands to reason there may be some confusion about what the Vagus nerve is doing in the social engagement system specifically. The internal organs of your body are connected to the brain by the connection created by the activated myelinated Vagus nerve, which is activated with the use of the social engagement system. Many of the other cranial nerves are associated with the face and neck. The Vagus nerve, on the other hand, is connected to the internal organs, which many people would not necessarily consider part of the social engagement system. But your internal organs and their impacted body parts need to know if there is a threat or not, so they can respond appropriately. For instance, in a secure state, your body relaxes its internal systems, allowing digestion to operate at a stable level, the heart to beat at a relaxed rate, the breath can slow, etc. But when there is a threat, it all changes. This activity created in your body is called the "vagal tone." This primarily deals with the amount of blood moving from the Vagus nerve to the various organs in your body it impacts. An engaged system allows the Vagus nerve to "talk" to the parts of the body through the passage of blood, meaning there is a high vagal tone.

The easiest place to observe this process is in the heart. The sinoatrial node is made of cells that are a natural regulator for your heart rate. The cells in this node are responsible for your rhythmic heart rate. Left unchecked, the rate of this heartbeat is much faster than your body needs while at rest. Left alone, the pace is about 110 beats per minute, while a resting heart rate for a healthy adult is between 60 and 80 beats per minute. To help stabilize this and relax the body through the heart rate the vagal tone is inhibiting this "pacemaker." It is called the "vagal brake" in this situation because it is responsible for slowing the heart rate down. It is like driving a car. You can "floor" the gas pedal but the car will only move forward if you release the brake. One of the "side effects" of this vagal brake is that when you slow the heart rate down you end up inhaling at a faster rate than you exhale. Take a moment to observe your breath now. Do you inhale quickly and then have a longer time to allow the oxygen to circulate in your body before it is fully released? Chances are you have a longer exhale. This makes your resting heart "rhythm" more of a variable and labeled as "arrhythmic." There is a correlation between the variability of your heart rate and your vagal tone. This means that you can observe the variability in your heart rate as a measure of your vagal tone as well.

This how the body responds when it is resting and there is no perceived threat. But what happens when it senses something? When this "threat" is detected, the sympathetic system is activated, inhibiting the social engagement system. This means your myelinated Vagus nerve is much less active and there is a drop in the vagal tone amount. This means less inhibition on the heart rate, allowing it to beat faster with a stronger rhythm. This then moves your blood around your body faster, moving oxygen and sugar at a faster clip. When your vagal tone drops like this it is called "vagal suppression." It is like lifting your foot up from the brake so the car can go.

There is a hierarchy to the neural control stages outlined. The most often used stage is the use of the myelinated Vagus nerve because it encourages a relaxed body with little energy use. This allows your behavior to more social and uses less of your internal "resources" to function. This, in turn, promotes growth and overall health. But when there is a threat or perceived threat, your internal "resources" are used to support your "fight, flight, or freeze" response instead of promoting cortical processing. This is why you may find it hard to remember things from a stressful moment or why you're thinking is muddled in extremely stressful situations. This is the activation of the sympathetic-adrenal system. And if the situation is extreme enough, the third stage, immobilization, can be activated.

It is important to recognize there is a difference between the three stages and what happens when they are activated. When you recognize why your body is responding a certain way it is easier to handle stressors and avoid negative health issues, like developing chronic stress. Moving from one stage to another is a normal process and something you probably do a few times a week or month. It is an evolutionary process that is designed to help you survive and even thrive. Left unchecked; however, it can lead to poor health conditions. You do not want to be switching again and again in a day. Responding to stress daily or multiple times a day is hard on your body. Now with this understanding and introduction to the polyvagal theory, you have the tools to recognize various illnesses and create coping methods to support your body and Vagus nerve.

Chapter 8: The Polyvagal Theory

The name of the Polyvagal Theory derives from "many" and "vagus nerve," and it embraces theoretical connection that is believed to exist between visceral or facial experiences and expressions, and physiological effects. These responses are mediated by the vagus nerve and purport to affect the digestive tract, the lungs and the heart. This effect is called **parasympathetic control.** Initial reactions to this theory, which was first presented by its originator, Dr. Stephen Porges, then at the University of Illinois, in 1994, evoked some skepticism, but over time and with extensive testing, the theory has been gaining traction. Today, serious research continues on the relationship between behavioral influences and their physiological effects.

The Impact Of Afferent Influences

Expression of the Polyvagal Theory is part of a larger scope called afferent influences bodily experiences and reactions that send impulses to the brain (as compared to efferent influences, which originate in the brain and flow outward). For example, a facial expression may influence the lungs by sending an **afferent** signal to the brain, which then sends an **efferent** signal to the lungs, directly affecting breathing rates. In practice, the theory is being applied to alleviate a range of physical disorders, such as bradycardia (slow heart rate), tachycardia (racing heart rate) and emotional disorders, including posttraumatic stress disorder (PTSD).

Related to these studies and practices is the conscious application of physical influences on one part of the body to another; for example, touching or rubbing the abdomen to send an afferent signal to the brain, and generating an efferent message that causes a slower heart rate or breathing rate.

Physical Reactions To Facial Expressions

The first step in studying the physiological effects of facial expressions is an assessment of how an individual's own facial expressions are influenced by the facial expressions of others. Studies confirm that exposure to certain facial expression evokes reactions in emotionally-reactive facial muscles of the person being observed. Many of the reactions are an emulation of the expressions they are seeing: a smile seen evokes a smile; a frown seen evokes a frown; a grimace evokes a grimace. The results conclude that there are definite correlations between facial expressions seen and evoked; these reactions occur on a subconscious level and include both negative and positive reactions.

One of Dr. Porges' discoveries is a previously unrecognized neural circuit, responsible for controlling facial muscles (and other muscles in the head); and capable of evoking emotional reactions in others. He named this the "social engagement system," and it states that when a person is in a relaxed state, their facial expressions and other bodily states can invite other people to feel relaxed and connected. This leads to the conclusion that if a person wants to connect with others, they should display a relaxed face, chest, and abdominal area.

Eye Contact: Physiological Support Of Responses

Eye contact has long been recognized as a way of either attracting or intimidating others. In a positive situation, eye contact, in association with a relaxed face, a smile or other encouraging expression can lead to a comfort level, forming a bond of common interest or attraction. In contrast, the confrontational act of "staring someone down" can have a powerful effect on driving a person away or evoking a conflict.

Now, there is physiological evidence to support at least the positive effects of mutually appealing eye contact. Studies show that our inner sense of stability and even positivity can influence the extent to which looking into another's eyes can release the hormone oxytocin, encouraging bonding in both participants. Alternatively, people experiencing stress, fear, or anger can stimulate stress hormones, diminishing the potential for cooperation when making eye contact.

The Polyvagal Theory, and other concepts that correlate physical and emotional responses to afferent influences, are supported in part by research into direct stimulation of the vagus nerve. These stimuli may be manual, or as needed in more serious medical situations, electrical.

There are potential applications of the more promising Polyvagal Theory findings on the commercial and military levels.

Commercial applications can adapt new facial recognition technologies that use artificial intelligence (AI) to distinguish facial attributes and characteristics to determine gender, age, ethnicity, as well as to recognize previously encountered individuals. For example, in a shopping mall, a facial-recognition camera embedded in an electronic advertising sign can instantly react and change its image, headline and key benefit claims to match the demographics of someone approaching the sign. In less than a second, the sign can present a young Asian woman's image to the approaching young woman of the same ethnicity.

Now, based on Polyvagal Theory findings, it may become possible for facial recognition software to "read" the facial expression of the approaching shopper, determine the mood or receptivity and attempt to make eye contact, image to person. The advertiser's objective would be to create a common bond, a sense of identification that can, in principle, increase the shopper's sense of identity with the advertised brand. In situations where the approaching shopper generates a negative or non-receptive countenance, the software could switch the advertisement to a more amusing, or curiosity-evoking image, potentially warming up the shopper's attitude.

Military and governmental applications of Polyvagal Theory findings are considerable. In meetings between politicians and their opponents, a hidden facial recognition camera could provide deeper insight into an opponent's true intentions. For example, is an offer being made with sincerity, with hope for a common agreement or is the opponent being deceptively charming, disguising different intentions. Behind the scenes, data from the hidden facial recognition camera can inform a staff member of the findings, and, when necessary, who can alert the politician via Bluetooth, of the real intentions, enabling a change of negotiating strategy.

The military applications can be similar to the governmental politicians' example, but in a different scenario, for example, a meeting with enemies across a negotiating table. "Can I trust him?" "Is this someone I can work with, constructively?" "Is the offer being made to me done so in sincerity?" Answers to these essential questions are normally determined judgmentally; now facial gestures, eye contacts (or the absence of) can more effectively measure intent.

In addition to the commercial, governmental and military applications, facial recognition software, enhanced with AI to read expressions and eye movements, can be of direct value in recruitment, more accurately assessing a candidate's willingness to "connect and bond."

Chapter 9: Vagus Nerve – An Introduction

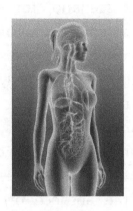

The vagus nerve serves as the cycle route of the body, transporting information between the brain and the internal organs, and controlling the response of the body during rest times. The large nerve comes from the brain and branches out to the neck and torso in multiple directions, where it is responsible for transporting sensory information from the skin of the ear, controlling the muscles you use to ingest, and speak and influencing your immune system.

According to the Encyclopedia Britannica, the vagus is the 10th of 12 cranial nerves, which extends directly from the brain. While we ascribe to the vagus nerve as singular, it is a pair of nerves that arise from the left and right side of the brain stem's fraction of the medulla oblongata. According to Merriam-Webster, which is appropriate, the nerve gets its name from the Latin word for wandering, since the vagus nerve is the largest and most widely branching cranial nerve.

The vagus nerve provides the primary control for the parasympathetic division of the nervous system, by roaming and venturing throughout the body: the rest-and-digest counterpoint to the fight-or-flight response of the sympathetic nervous system. The vagus nerve sends directives that slow heart and respiration levels and boost digestion when the body is not under stress—control shifts to the sympathetic system in times of stress that generates the reverse effect.

The vagus nerve also carries sensory signals back into the brain from internal organs, allowing the brain to keep a record of the actions of the organs.

1.1 Branches

Auricular nerve

Pharyngeal nerve

Superior laryngeal nerve

Superior cervical cardiac branches of the vagus nerve

Inferior cervical cardiac branch

Recurrent laryngeal nerve

Thoracic, cardiac branch

Branch to the pulmonary plexus

Branch to the esophageal plexus

Anterior vagal trunk

Posterior vagal trunk

Herring Breuer reflux in alveoli

The vagus leads posterior to the common carotid artery and internal jugular vein inside the carotid sheath.

1.2 Innervation

The right and left nerves of the vagus descend from the brain in the carotid sheath, vertically to the carotid artery. The right nerve of the vagus leads to the right recurrent laryngeal nerve that hooks around the right subclavian artery and ascends between the trachea and the esophagus into the neck.

Then the right vagus crosses the right subclavian artery anteriorly and runs back to the upper vena cava and descends back to the right main bronchus and contributes to cardiac, respiratory, and esophageal plexus. It creates the posterior vagal trunk at the bottom of the esophagus and passes through the esophageal hiatus into the diaphragm.

The left vagus nerve enters the thorax in between the left carotid artery and the left subclavian artery and descends into the aortic arch. It gives rise to the recurrent left laryngeal nerve that hooks to the left of the ligamentum arteriosum around the aortic arch and ascends between the trachea and esophagus.

Furthermore, the left vagus gives off thoracic, cardiac branches, breaks up into the pulmonary plexus, proceeds into the esophageal plexus, and enters the belly as the anterior vagal trunk in the diaphragm's esophageal hiatus. The vagus nerve supplies all organs with parasympathetic motor fibers except for the suprarenal (adrenal) glands, from the neck down to the second tran segment.

1.3 Muscles controlled by Vagus Nerve

The vagus also controls some skeletal muscles, i.e.

Cricothyroid muscle

Levator veli palatini muscle

Salpingopharyngeal muscle

Palatopharyngeal muscle

Supreme, middle and inferior pharyngeal constrictors

Laryngeal muscles (speech).

It implies that perhaps the vagus nerve is personally liable for such diverse tasks as heart rate, gastrointestinal peristalsis, sweating, and very a few muscle movements in the mouth including speech (through the recurrent laryngeal nerve) and holding the larynx open for respiration (through movement of the posterior cricoarytenoid muscle, the only abductor of the vocal folds). And it has some afferent fibers that internalize the inner (channel) portion of the outer ear, through the Auricular branch (also known as the nerve of Alderman) and part of the meninges. This describes why a person may be coughing on his or her ear (such as removing ear wax with a cotton swab).

1.4 The vagus nerve and the heart

The vagus nerve is mediated by parasympathetic innervation of the heart. The vagus nerve merely serves to decrease the heart rate. The right vagus innervates the sinoatrial node. Parasympathetic hyperstimulation predisposes all infected to bradyarrhythmias. The left vagus, when hyper stimulated, influences the blocks of the heart to atrioventricular (AV). Neuroscientist Otto Loewi first proved at this place that nerves secrete substances called neurotransmitters with effects on receptors throughout the target tissue. Loewi identified the content produced by the vagus nerve as vagusstoff, later found to be acetylcholine. The vagus nerve has three nuclei associated with cardiovascular regulation in the CNS, the dorsal motor nucleus, the uncertain nucleus, and the solitary nucleus. The parasympathetic contribution to the heart comes primarily from neurons in the ambiguous nucleus and, to a minimal extent, from the dorsal motor nucleus. The isolated nucleus provides sensory feedback about the condition of the cardiovascular system as an integrated channel for the baroreflex. Drugs that suppress the cholinergic muscarinic receptor (anticholinergic receptor) such as atropine and scopolamine are called vagolytic.

1.5 What affects occurs by Vagus Nerve?

The vagus nerve has different features. The vagus nerve's four main functions are:

Sensory: From the throat, heart, lungs, and abdomen.

Special sensory: Provides a sense of taste behind the tongue.

Motor: Provides movement functions for the neck muscles responsible for swallowing and speaking.

Parasympathetic: Responsible for the operation of the digestion tract, respiration, and heart rate.

Its functions can be further broken down into seven groups. Each of these is the nervous system working itself. We Can split the nervous system into two areas: sympathetic and parasympathetic. The side of sympathy increases alertness, stamina,

blood pressure, heart rate, and respiration rate. The parasympathetic part, which actively includes the vagus nerve, reduces alertness, blood pressure, and heart rate, and assists with calmness, relaxation, and digestion. The vagus nerve, therefore, also deals with defecation, urination, and sexual arousal.

Many vagus nerve effects include:

Brain-to-intestinal communication: the vagus nerve sends input to the brain from the gut.

Deep breath relaxation: The nerve vagus interacts with the diaphragm. An individual feels more relaxed with deep breaths.

Decrease Inflammation: The vagus nerve provides an anti-inflammatory signal to other parts of the body.

Diminishing heart rate and blood pressure: If the vagus nerve is overactive, the heart may not pump blood around the body. In some cases, excessive activity of the nerve vagus may cause loss of consciousness and damage to the organ.

Fear management: The vagus nerve sends information from the intestine to the brain that is linked to stress, anxiety, and fear – hence the saying, "good feeling." These signals help a person recover from stressful and frightening situations.

Chapter 10: The Power Of Your Mind And Your Healing System

Your mind is your healing system's most powerful ally. Working through your brain and nervous system, your mind can send powerful messages to your body that can dramatically influence the performance of your healing system. Through these mechanisms, a sophisticated communication feedback system sends precise, split-second information from your body back to your brain. Your mind remains in intimate contact with your body's ever-changing internal environment while it works side by side with your healing system. In the words of well-known physician and author Dr. Andrew Weil, "Wherever nerves are, activities of the mind can travel."

All mental activity, whether conscious or unconscious, has a powerful influence on your healing system and can enhance or interfere with its performance. For example, when your mind is in a positive state, immersed in thoughts of love and affection, caring and compassion, enthusiasm, health, happiness, joy, and peace, beneficial chemicals known as neurotransmitters or neuropeptides that are secreted by your brain can actually infuse your body with positive energy, strengthening your healing system and improving your health. Alternatively, when your mind is in a negative state, with thoughts of pessimism, cynicism, jealousy, anger, hatred, fear, revenge, self-criticism, blame, shame, guilt, and despair, you are sending negative messages to your body via equally powerful chemicals that can weaken your healing system and interfere with its ability to do its job effectively. In the words of Robert Eliot, M.D., "The brain writes prescriptions for the body."

When you understand the power of your mind, and its enormous ability to work either for you or against you, you will no longer waste valuable time or energy blaming outside forces, including rate, bad genes, evil microbes, a polluted environment, or other people for your illnesses, diseases, or lack of good health. Outside forces can certainly play a role in disease processes, but, in the final analysis, your health is based more on the personal choices you make for yourself, moment by moment, each day of your life, and your ability to optimize the incredible power of your mind to aid your healing system. You are the one who is ultimately responsible for your health, and so it is imperative that you understand this principle. More than any other power or force in this world, your own mind can serve as your healing system's most qualified and capable partner.

Mind as Healer, Mind as Killer

You can use your mind for your body's ultimate health and healing, or you can use it in a way that turns against you to the detriment of your health. Your mind and your thoughts can cause real physiological changes in your body, as the placebo effect demonstrates. If you learn to use your mind to cooperate with your body's healing system, it can be your healing system's most powerful ally, a loyal servant and friend. If you do not use them properly, your mind and thoughts, through the release of powerful neuropeptides, hormones, and electrical nerve stimulation, can weaken and damage your body's health, interfere with your healing system, and cause premature physical deterioration, disease, and even your ultimate demise. If it is not properly trained and used, your mind can become a definite liability, prove to be your worst enemy, and even kill you.

Infusing Your Healing System with Positive Beliefs

Beliefs are powerful thoughts that we hold onto and invest with great energy as if they were true, even though they might not be true. Your beliefs help to shape the way you think and view the world, and often they are backed by the collective support of many people, including family and friends. Your beliefs are also reinforced and influenced by many factors, including your education, the books you read, the media, your colleagues, peers, community, religious preferences, gender, and age, and your own personal thoughts and unique life experiences.

Beliefs can be passed down from one generation to the next. They can extend far back in time, covering centuries, and even millennia. Beliefs often gain strength over time. The more people who share in a similar, common belief, the more powerful that belief becomes. 'When beliefs become heavily invested with a lot of time and energy, letting go of them and changing them is difficult, even when they are wrong. For example, in medieval Europe, before Christopher Columbus's historic voyage in 1492, the belief was that the world was flat, and that if you sailed too far out to sea, you would fall off the edge of the world, Of course, we now know that this belief was not true, but for hundreds of years, many peoples' lives were affected by this limited view.

Beliefs are constructed of powerful thoughts, and as such, they can play a major role in determining your health. Beliefs can significantly influence the performance of your body's healing system through the powerful messages they send to every organ, tissue, and cell in your body. If your beliefs are positive, healthy, and life-sustaining, they can work to your advantage. For example, in a well-known study that looked at Harvard University graduates over a 25-year period, those who believed their health was good or excellent at the beginning of the study had significantly fewer illnesses and diseases, far better survival statistics, and reported enjoying much better health at the end of the 25-year study period

than those who reported their health as
only fair or poor.

Emotions and Your Healing System

Emotions are packets of mental and
physical energy that move through and
attempt to move out of your body, much
like a river whose water steadily moves
toward its greater destiny of the ocean.
The word emotion comes from the root
emote, which means to move out.

Your emotions have a profound impact on
your physical health, and they play an
integral role in the functioning of your
healing system. Your emotions are
connected to your endocrine system,
which includes your pineal, pituitary,
thyroid, parathyroid, and adrenal glands,
as well as your pancreas and reproductive
organs.

During emotional experiences, powerful
hormones are released into your
bloodstream from these various organs,
and these hormones have far-reaching

effects on your body and your healing system. For example, when you are in a highly excitable state, either feeling exuberant joy or intense fear, your adrenal glands release epinephrine (adrenaline), which can constrict blood vessels, accelerate heart rate, increase blood pressure, and affect lung and kidney function. Cortisol, which can suppress your immune function, is also released at these times. All of these functions are critical to your healing system. Insulin, which regulates sugar metabolism, is also produced in response to certain emotions, especially when you are feeling frightened, angry, or under stress. These are just a few of the more commonly known hormones associated with your emotions, but you can see what a profound effect they can have on your healing system.

Being in touch with your feelings, understanding what they are and what they mean, is important for the health of your healing system. When you are in touch with how you feel, you usually feel energized and alive. When you are out of touch with your emotions, you tend to feel separated from life, isolated and lonely. Feelings of loneliness and isolation create stress, which, if sustained, can have harmful repercussions on your healing system.

Clear evidence now exists that suppressing emotions can be damaging to your health and your body's healing system. Repressing emotions goes against the natural laws of the universe that require the natural energy of emotions to move out of your body to seek conscious expression. Numerous studies have shown that people who continuously suppress their emotions are more likely to fall prey to serious illnesses, including heart disease, hypertension, diabetes, cancer, autoimmune diseases, and other chronic conditions.

Other studies have shown that people who are able to access their feelings and express themselves enjoy better health and greater longevity. Rather than suppressing your feelings and emotions, most medical experts are now recommending that to prevent illness, it is important to get in touch with your feelings, whatever they are, and then learn to express them in healthy ways.

Healthy feelings create sensations of comfort and ease in your body. Some healthy feelings are joy, happiness, peace, contentment, serenity, satisfaction, and love. Because they release powerful hormones, these feelings are extremely beneficial to the health of your body's internal environment, and they can keep your healing system vibrant and strong for many years. Of course, the most powerful healthy feeling of all is love.

Because feelings are located in our bodies, there are really no negative feelings or emotions, though this probably sounds like a contradiction. Feelings just are, and they cannot be judged on any level by anyone. Even anger, pain, and sadness, generally considered to be "negative" emotions, can be appropriate and beneficial, especially when we acknowledge and release them from our bodies in a timely and sensible manner. The problem occurs when we do not release these emotions, but rather, as we discussed before, we hold onto and contain or suppress them. Under these circumstances, suppression of so-called negative emotions can be harmful. Healing often occurs when the roots of these unhealthy emotions are exposed and then released from your body.

Chapter 11: What Happens When The Vagus Nerve Isn't Operating Well?

A small amount of research into the vagus nerve reveals a whole array of disorders that have either been positively correlated or are currently being investigated for a connection to the nerve. We vary from minor annoyances to major issues. Of course, if you're influenced anywhere in the continuum, it can impact your overall sense of well-being and overall performance.

Some people will experience a vasovagal response at some point due to a stressor or overstimulation of the vagus nerve. Blood pressure drops, the heart rate increases and the blood vessels in your legs expand, which can induce discomfort or fainting. It is usually a benign reaction that continues on its own, although those individuals who feel it more frequently may need to pursue professional help.

Many problems related to vagus nervous disease include hypertension, nausea, mood disorders, bradycardia, gastrointestinal disorders, chronic inflammation, fainting, and epilepsy.

Of course, any of these factors may contribute to more illnesses, such as obesity and inflammation, all related to cancer and diabetes. Anxiety or mood disorders may also lead to depression.

How Does The "Hacking" Of The Vagus Work?

There is a growing body of research indicating that we can exploit or "attack" the vagus nerve. Vagus hackers date back to work done by Kevin Tracey in 1998. Via his research, he found that he could reduce the inflammatory response of the body by activating the vagus nerve with an electrical impulse.

It had a beneficial impact on the diagnosis of illnesses such as Crohn's disease, rheumatoid arthritis and other infectious diseases. Tracey's work formed the foundation for the theory of bioelectronics, which we now see as managing disorders such as depression and epilepsy.

Regardless of such conditions, inflammation is a reaction that we all have in our bodies, mostly due to stress. For some individuals (here, entrepreneurs!), depression and allergic responses can become recurrent, contributing to other health problems.

The vagus nerve is connected to so many different functions that there are more "hacks" than the bioelectric system inserted to activate it (usually only in extreme cases). In reality, researchers have found that we can combat inflammation by stimulating the vagus nerve and enhancing the "vagal tone"–

kind of like a workout! Let's look at what you can do:

1. You focus on your emotional health

A 2010 study found that a strong vagal tone was part of the feedback loop between physical health, positive emotions, and positive social interactions. For a self-sustaining dynamic, these variables affect each other.

During the trial, the researchers used Loving Kindness Meditation (LKM) as a means to positively influence their emotional health. Studies had found that when people focused on positive social interactions or worked to improve their interaction with other people, they had a beneficial effect on the vagal tone.

Take-away: to engage in activities that promote positive feelings and social connections. Yoga, yoga, relaxation, and connecting with others can improve.

2. Focus on the wellbeing of the heart

Do you realize the "good feeling" is a true thing? Signals from the vagus nerve are passing from the stomach to the cortex. This has been related to a modulating attitude and to certain forms of fear and anxiety. A hallmark of a good vagal tone is someone who has grace under pressure–a quality that most businessmen could use!

Your vagus nerve is continuously transmitting up-to-date sensory input about the status of your body's organs, digestive tract, heart rate, and other details to your brain through various nerves. Research shows that our intestinal bacteria and the pathways to the brain are interlinked. The intestinal microbiota is also considered to be the possible primary modulator of the immune and nervous systems. Maintaining a healthy intestine is, therefore, an ambiguous ' fix.' Take-away: good health varies from person to person and depends on how you are made, but in general, you can: take probiotics, eat a healthy, balanced diet of whole grains, avoid unnecessary use of antibiotics, and moderate consumption of sugary foods or alcohol. In fact, although probiotics are still being studied for their effectiveness, a Canadian study found them to be successful in PTSD care. There are also consequences for the management of depression—discovering whether you can benefit from taking them can be a simple step forward.

3. Use the breathing technique

Breathing techniques also entered Western awareness sometime around the 1970s, but Eastern people have been using such methods for centuries. It turns out there is sound science behind deep breathing —you can help activate the vagus nerve and increase the amplitude of the heart rate (HRV).

Chapter 12: How Vagus Nerve Helps Control Your Anger

Allowing yourself to consciously express the anger you feel is very healthy, not only emotionally, but also physically. Repressed anger makes people sick. It causes a person to turn their anger toward themselves. This pent-up anger usually leads to people feeling drained and depressed. The problem is that we haven't been really taught how to express our emotions in a healthy manner, which is why we often end up stuffing all our feelings inside, especially anger.

On the contrary, we have been taught to avoid anger and other feelings related to it. But if you come to think of it, our emotions, including anger, are there for a reason. Instead of going against your anger when you're feeling like you want to explode, decide to go with the flow. But then again, make sure you know how to safely express your anger, so that you avoid hurting other people and avoid hurting yourself.

Anger is an extremely potent emotion that can originate from any multitude of feelings such as disappointment, sadness, hurt, resentment, etc. It's a standard emotion that everyone has felt and that everyone feels differently, whether they are mildly annoyed or enraged. It's natural to feel anger no matter what the strength of that anger is. Anger can range from minor irritation to steady frustration, to blind rage. Any amount of anger a person feels should be validated, just as a person's depression, anxiety, happiness, etc. should be. Anger is not just an emotional response, but it is also a physical response within the body. When you begin to feel angry, your body produces extra adrenaline and cortisol, which are "stress hormones." This causes your blood to travel faster to the muscles in your arms and legs in order to allow your body to physically react fast enough to avoid the threat that it recognizes your anger as. This causes less blood in your brain, causing the thought process to become "cloudy." So, while you are feeling your anger mentally, the rest of your body is feeling it too.

Anger can be caused by multiple things internally or externally. Things like negative thought patterns are an internal stimulus that can cause anger, while an external stimulus could be something happening due to another person that is outside of your control. Indeed, anger can essentially be referred to as a moral emotion due to it coming forward in times of injustice against oneself or others. Though justified in those types of situations, it can cause a person to go too far with their defense when they are not under control. Without techniques or a plan to control yourself when you are feeling angry, your anger can become a big problem.

Using anger as a coping mechanism is not a healthy way to approach any sort of problem and can lead to it becoming too much to handle. When anger goes uncontrolled it can have a harmful effect on the person feeling it, in addition to the other people that interact with them. The effect it has on mental health can lead to more problematic issues like strained romantic or familial relationships, strained friendships, poor work performance, poor academic performance, etc. In some extremes, it can even lead to more serious problems or actions such as physical abuse, emotional abuse, substance abuse, and other criminal activity due to the lack of impulse control and aggression that can result from untreated anger problems. Aggression is the feeling of actually wanting to cause harm to someone physically or mentally, so when a person's anger is building up within them, they may start to act out aggressively toward others and hurt someone else or themselves. That is the main reason that anger needs to be under control, to prevent anyone from being hurt.

When it goes unmanaged, it focuses more on the emotional moment and the perceived problem rather than finding a solution. This is another reason why managing it is important, because you may feel less stressed and have better problem-solving skills in the long run. Anger is also connected with the concept of the instincts fight, flight, and freeze. Anger is one of the driving forces behind the "fight" instinct, meaning that anger allows your brain and body to choose fighting as an option when it is necessary in times of self-preservation. This is an important reason that anger should be regulated within everyone so that their brains and bodies stay alert and are able to be stimulated when necessary, rather than in times that you are lacking control of yourself.

Chronic, unmanaged anger has been linked to many different health complications;

Digestive issues

High blood pressure

Skin problems

Joint pain

Insomnia

Dizziness/lightheadedness

Ulcers

Strokes

Hormonal imbalances

Chronic headaches

An increase in anxiety levels

Depression

Hypertension

Eczema and other skin conditions

Heart attack

When all of these different physical reactions are happening at a frequent rate, it can possibly lead to permanent physical problems when left non-maintained. When someone is having some, or even all, of these physical and mental ailments due to anger, that means it has started to dominate their life and needs to be addressed.

While learning to cope with your anger can help many of these conditions to disappear, the long-term damage may already be done in some cases and it can take you much longer to heal. Looking at the last condition, how many people actually realize that frequent bouts of anger can exponentially raise their risks of a heart attack?

How Is the Vagus Nerve is Involved in dealing with Anger?

The vagus nerve is responsible for managing the relaxed state in which people are able to rest. However, just as with anger, when the vagus nerve is unable to trigger the parasympathetic nervous system to rule the body, the sympathetic nervous system is allowed to reign supreme over the body, wreaking its havoc as it continues for too long. The vagus nerve, of course, is going to be sending impulses back to your brain to fill it in with how the body is feeling, due to its afferent status. The longer this anger goes on as well, the less likely it is that the parasympathetic nervous system will kick into play in the first place, meaning that you will be less likely to be able to defeat that anger at any given point in time. Unless you are able to kick-start your vagus nerve back in gear to get it moving, you are going to struggle.

Exercises to Stimulate the Vagus Nerve to Combat Anger Symptoms

A common technique used in managing anger is taking slow and deep breaths. The mechanism behind this is that deep breathing activates the vagus nerve and enables it to restore the body to a relaxed and rested state. This is crucial when it comes to stress management. People with poor vagal activity are prone to chronic stress and depressive tendencies because their fight and flight response system are not being sufficiently kept in check by the vagus nerve.

Scream Inside Your Room

While it's still unclear what effects screaming will have on the individual, it's certain that many people believe such practice is a great way to let your emotions out. If you're going to scream, though, see to it that you do it inside your room and with your face covered as screaming may have negative effects on those who hear it.

Exercise

Anger is normally a result of frustration and anxiety and countless studies have shown that exercise relieves anxiety and depression.

Physical exercise also burns off the excess energy and releases endorphins into the blood that lift your mood, hence the term, "runners high". It reduces blood pressure, which is also a factor in anger, be it the cause or a result.

Breathing Therapy

One of the most prominent techniques in anger management is teaching ways to control your breathing in a way that assists in de-escalating anger. These deep breathing exercises can act as a momentary distraction. It's actually more than just a distraction, it's the reversal of your body's biological response to angry feelings. Controlled breathing in situations of anger sends a signal through the body to help it begin to calm after the release of adrenalin sent through the body. It also helps the body return to a balanced level of carbon dioxide and oxygen, rather than the unbalanced levels that happen when the body is feeling tension.

Massage Therapy

Massage is generally seen as a way of relaxing and "chilling out" as well as treating specific issues, such as pain, range of movement, etc.

Massage therapy can also help you to sleep better at night, which leaves you feeling more rested and able to cope with whatever the day throws at you without resorting to angry outbursts. Regular massage therapy is a good idea for anyone who struggles with anger and is prone to emotional outbursts.

Meditate to Relax your Mind

You will eventually learn to worry only about what is important and let the small stuff get away, reliving your mind of tension, worry and anxiety.

Meditation is one of the more powerful forms of holistic treatment. When you get angry or stressed out, your adrenal glands secrete cortisol – the angrier you get, the more cortisol is released and this leads to tight muscles, hypertension, racing heart and a surge of adrenaline. Meditation works by rebalancing the cortisol, giving your body a much-needed break and the ability to think more clearly.

Meditation also helps to melt away feelings of stress, anxiety and depression, all of which are causes of anger. It teaches you how to be the master of your emotions and it raises your threshold for stress, making it less likely that you will lose your temper and succumb to the dark energy of anger.

The third benefit of meditation is that it boosts the production of serotonin in your body. Serotonin is known as the "feel good" hormone and, when it is released, it produces feeling of euphoria and happiness, creating a high state of awareness and leaving you feeling much cooler and calmer.

Pray, Smile and Keep Faith

Prayer is one of the best forms of support and reassurance that can help to keep you free from anxiety. Developing a habit of praying and chanting daily can help to fill you with positive energy, help to calm the mind and instill a sense of faith that the world and all in it is taken care of by a higher power. Also, make an effort to smile more often, as it will make you feel happier and instill you with a sense of confidence and positivity.

Sing or Dance

Singing or dancing in itself won't get rid of the anger you're feeling inside. Moreover, when you're doing creative things like dancing or singing, it's almost impossible to fix your mind on other things--your anger, for instance--since you're focused on what you're doing. Singing and dancing can help you be fully in the present and help you welcome distractions from the issues of life at the same time.

Chapter 13: Stress, Inflammation, And Vagal Tone

In case you haven't realized it by now, many aspects of the mental health discussion above were related to stress. Anxiety causes a stressful response. Trauma reactions are often literally severe stress reactions. And depression causes a different type of stress that makes us want to shut down. All of these reactions result in a more suppressed vagus nerve, which means that we remain in a state of alertness. Our sympathetic nervous system stays active long after it should shut off. Knowing how to activate the vagus nerve can help us reduce our stress responses in so many different kinds of situations. Because stress is involved in inflammation and poor sleep habits, we'll discuss all three in this chapter. We'll also discuss how our body reacts to these situations and how activating the ventral vagus nerve can help us reduce our stress and inflammation while improving our sleep.

Stress

Imagine that you're at work, plugging away and completing what you're supposed to. Suddenly your boss sends you a message requesting that you complete these other items by the end of the day. You can handle it, so you take on those additional tasks. Within the next few minutes, you realize that they're a whole lot larger than you thought they were going to be, so you start to feel overwhelmed. Maybe an hour later, your child's school calls, saying that little Kate is sick and needs to go home. Suddenly you have a full plate with work and a sick child to care for, and your original feeling of being overwhelmed is now a full-blown feeling of being stressed.

Your body starts to release all of these hormones that increase your feelings of stress. Your blood pressure rises, your heart rate increases, and your muscles get tense. This is your sympathetic nervous system coming online to help you deal with the dangerous situation. However, there isn't any actual danger, just a lot of work. Your brain, though, sees this situation as dangerous and puts you in the beginning stages of fight or flight, causing your ventral vagus nerve to retreat. Eventually, once your work is completed and little Kate is better, your brain will tell your ventral vagus that the threat has passed, and your vagus nerve will hit the brakes on your stress response, giving you feelings of calm and well-being, while reducing your heart rate and breathing rate.

This feeling is probably familiar to you. You may not even be aware of the changes in your physiology until you've been stressed for a while. By that point, you've been operating in a high alert state for a bit and then need your vagus nerve to step in. But if your brain still thinks there's a threat, then it won't. The fact is that your body will reactivate its sympathetic nervous system again and again anytime it perceives a threat, including just feeling overwhelmed at work. This frequent activation of being always on alert can do damage to your body. Your heart can start to feel strain, your hormones can cause your blood pressure to remain high, and you are at more risk for cardiovascular issues and obesity. If you experience high amounts of stress every day, then this is how your body responds to it.

Inflammation

Inflammation is when your body decides that it needs to protect itself from attack. This could be from diseases, bacteria, or wounds. You're probably already familiar with experiencing inflammation. If you've ever had a cut on your body, you will have noticed how the area turned red and was painful. This was your body's natural inflammatory response to help heal your body after the wound. It doesn't matter how big or small your wound is, your body tries to heal it through inflammation. You would have also experienced inflammation whenever you've been sick with the flu or similar disease. Your body responds to diseases by increasing your body temperature, flaring up pain signals, and sending white blood cells to combat whatever is causing the issue. While all of this is to your benefit since it can help with healing, too much inflammation can also be very negative.

Having too much of an inflammatory response means that your body starts to focus on areas that either don't need healing or do, but the inflammation causes the problems to worsen. This results in chronic, debilitating pain. Rheumatoid arthritis is one example of a severe inflammatory response that does more damage than good. Perhaps, unsurprisingly, having negative inflammatory responses can be triggered by stress.

Inflammation and stress go together hand-in-hand. Chronic stress can trigger your body to start an inflammatory response. When you're feeling stressed all the time, your body gets used to the hormones released and 'numb' to the ones released to help you heal. Because your body gets used to its stress hormones, it becomes less responsive to the inflammatory ones that are trying to heal it. This can lead to your body being more impacted by diseases. If your inflammatory response isn't working well because of stress, this means that you're more susceptible to colds, fevers, and diseases.

Because stress and inflammation are related, that means that you can work on them both by activating your vagus nerve. So if you reduce your stress by activating your vagus nerve, you'll also be able to reduce your inflammation. Surprisingly, scientists have found that implants that trigger stimulation of the vagus nerve do help with reduced inflammation, particularly with inflammation like arthritis. Stress and inflammation are both connected to your vagus nerve and vagal tone.

Vagal Tone

Vagal tone is how your vagus nerve is measured based on its connection with your heart rate. It is an indication of how well your vagus nerve is working. Your vagus nerve regulates your heart rate by slowing it down during your exhales. So as you inhale, your heart speeds up, and as you exhale, your heart slows down. This improves your vagal tone and reduces your blood pressure, makes you feel calm, and keeps you in that 'rest and digest stage.' Needless to say, anything that affects your heart will then affect your vagus nerve. And stress is a well-known disease that affects your heart.

Stress lowers your vagal tone or reduces the activation of your vagus nerve. Because this shifts your vagus nerve, it means that it also changes how your heart rate changes. This leads to you having a faster heart rate and an increase in physical illness. A lower vagal tone is associated with all of the mental struggles we discussed earlier, and it's also attached to cardiovascular disease, stroke, and more. So having a lower vagal tone is not the best for your body. Conversely, having a higher vagal tone results in you having better well-being.

Now you may be wondering why vagal tone is discussed here at this point of the book. The reason is this: By this point in the book, you should be able to see how everything is interconnected. Stress changes your vagal tone which changes your emotional regulation. Emotional regulation is part of the struggle of dealing with depression. Trauma creates a massive stress response to the environment, which lowers your vagal tone and results in your vagus nerve going into 'freeze' more often than it should, while also increasing your sympathetic nervous response. Anxiety is the same, as it causes stress which reduces your vagal tone, which in turn causes more anxiety. It's all interconnected in a cycle that keeps being perpetuated between your environment, brain, and vagus nerve. The only way to break the cycle is to activate your vagus nerve and improve your vagal tone. Every self-help technique discussed so far does this. In the next chapter, we are going to look at additional techniques that can help reduce your stress response and improve your vagal tone.

Chapter 14: Practical Self Help Exercises For Vagus Nerve Activation

Now that you know how the vagus nerve operates and why it is important for your health, let us now focus on its application. Many people are quick to use any means of vagus nerve activation that comes their way. As already mentioned, there are some techniques of vagus nerve activation that are helpful while others are harmful. You must be cautious not to use harmful techniques. Continuous activation of the vagus nerve using the wrong techniques may lead to chronic inflammation, which may be a source for more trouble. We have already looked at the negative effects associated with vagus nerve inflammation.

Breathing Techniques for Vagus Nerve Activation

To help activate the vagus nerve, you can adapt diaphragmatic breathing. In this type of breathing, the aim is to reduce the tension on the lungs and the heart. When you use this type of breathing, you allow yourself to take in air in slow bits that help reduce pressure. Diaphragmatic breathing helps in expanding the diaphragm. This is effective in reducing blood pressure and calming down nerves during anxious moments. The reduction of pressure and calming of nerves helps the body activate parasympathetic actions of the vagus nerve. The activation of parasympathetic action eventually leads to rest. Here is a step by step guide to diaphragmatic breathing.

Step 1: Position Yourself

When you want to breathe and calm down your nerves, you must align your body in a position that allows sufficient intake of air. In simple terms, your lungs should be open. If you try diaphragmatic breathing while you are lying on your belly or sitting in a bad position, you will strain; your body should be free enough to allow enough air into your lungs. The best positions include when you are standing upright or when you are seated upright. You can stand in an upright position and slightly spread your arms. This posture opens up your chest to allow sufficient air in. If you are seated on a chair or a mat, ensure that your back is in an upright position. This allows you to freely inhale the air.

Step 2: Inhale and Pause

After positioning yourself strategically, inhale a large chunk of air slowly and hold it in. You can hold your breath for about ten seconds or even more. Given that regular breathing includes 10 - 14 inhalations per minute, the diaphragmatic breathing usually involves around 6 inhalations per minute. When you inhale the fresh air, do not be in a hurry to let it out. Hold on to it for a few seconds; approximately 10, then release it gently.

Step 3: Slowly Exhale

After about ten seconds, you can now exhale and start the process all over. When you let out the air, you feel as if space has been freed up, and a weight has been lifted off your shoulders. The exhalation process helps clean your body of all negative energy. When you release the air, you allow your body to calm down and resume normal activities. It is important to note that this type of breathing should be well coordinated to work. If you do not allow yourself to calm down and try focusing on your breath, the effort may be worthless. As much as you want to enjoy your life and get rid of anxiety, you must try training your thoughts to focus on your breathing. You need to allow yourself to visualize the entire process.

Exercises That Activate Your Vagus Nerve

Exercising on a daily basis can also affect your vagus nerve. We know that physical activities are directly influential on your heart rate and blood pressure. These activities may moderate the heart rate or may increase it depending on your condition. While physical activities are effective in controlling the vagus nerve, not all activities will work out. In most cases, it is the gentle physical activities that do not require a lot of energy that works well in activating the vagus nerve. The two main physical activities used in vagus nerve activation include yoga and tai-chi.

Yoga: Yoga is a form of physical activity that involves stretching of the body muscles in combination with meditation and affirmation recitations. Yoga combines so many physiotherapeutic techniques in one session. If you want to benefit from the vagus nerve activation ability of yoga, you need to find the right yoga trainer. You can also perform yoga at home by using guided videos. One important factor to keep in mind when it comes to performing yoga is that the session should be mind calming. When performing yoga for vagus activation, try incorporating other techniques such as slow breathing, and meditation. To perform yoga well, you will need a quiet location with minimal disruptions. You will also need a yoga mat and a guide video. If you prefer performing among other individuals, you can get into a yoga studio around your home.

Tai-chi: Tai-chi is a form of wrestling technique originating from ancient China. The technique today is performed as a form of exercise. Tai-chi mainly involves slow horizontal movements with the hands placed in front of the practitioner. This type of exercise has been found to be calming and very helpful to individuals who wish to stimulate their vagus nerve. If you want to stimulate your vagus nerve, simply focus on working out on the slow movements. You can use a guided video to perform tai-chi, or you may choose to visit a studio near you.

Meditation for Vagus Nerve Activation

Meditation is one of the most important ways of activating the vagus nerve. Meditation can be used by any person, even those who have not attended meditation classes. As compared to tai-chi and yoga, which seem to be complex, meditation is a simple approach.

Meditation simply involves visualization. The practitioner has to visualize a certain environment that promotes calmness. The main aim of meditation in this process is to calm down the sympathetic action and activate the parasympathetic action of the vagus nerve. If you are capable of sending a signal to the brain that will initiate the actions of the parasympathetic nervous system, you will be in the right position to move on with your life.

To benefit from meditation, you need to choose the right type of meditation. There are many types of meditation. However, only a few are effective in calming down nerves and boosting your vagus nerve action. Some of the meditation techniques used to activate the vagus nerve include:

Mindfulness Meditation: In this type of meditation, the aim is to distract the mind from the thoughts that cause anxiety. When you practice mindfulness meditation, the focus is on yourself. You only think about yourself, your body, your environment, among others. If you want to enjoy the fruits of mindful meditation, you need to observe the rules for mindful meditation. First, during mindfulness, a person may discover some frustrating facts about themselves. In mindful meditation, you allow yourself to visualize yourself in a way that you have never done before. Therefore, all the benefits of the meditation should be protected by following the rules. One of the most important rules of this type of meditation is being non-judgmental. In other words, you are not allowed to judge yourself after observing your thoughts or feelings. You are required to embrace the truth about yourself. This action in itself promotes calming of nerves. Some people who suffer from depression only experience nervousness due to fear of being judged. However, if you can learn to accept your flaws through mindfulness meditation, you will not be shaken by anything. Mindfulness meditation teaches you to stand strong and believe in yourself no matter what the world may say about you. This is the attitude you need to overcome anxiety and depression. This attitude also promotes the parasympathetic activities of the vagus nerve.

Focused Meditation: Focused meditation is a type of meditation where the practitioner focuses their thoughts on a single object. In this type of meditation, you can choose any object in a room and simply focus on it. Focused meditation needs intense concentration. For instance, you can choose to focus on a chair or a wall. When performing focused meditation, you can't release your eyes from that piece of furniture. Use your mind to describe the chair and try looking at it based on different aspects. Think about its design, colors, shape, make, or any other aspect of the seat. Think about factors that make it special, how it holds weight, among others. This type of meditation is only intended to help you reduce the tension in your mind. After reducing the tension on your mind, the body can slowly reduce the sympathetic actions that are leading anxiety.

Peace, Love, and Kindness Meditation: This is the most ideal type of meditation for individuals looking to activate the vagus nerve. The fact that a person may be experiencing anxiety or depression means that they need an activity that will lead to the calming down of nerves. There is no better activity than peace, love, and kindness meditation.

In this type of meditation, you have to visualize yourself as a center of peace, love, and kindness to the world. In your mind, you have to visualize a world without violence or hatred. In this world, you are the main source of peace, love, and kindness. In this type of meditation, you visualize yourself extending kindness to people who need it. You stand out as an individual who embraces those who are weak. In your routines, you provide peace and kindness to people who are close to you and try to show them that the world can be a better place. You freely gift people who need help on the streets. You may also visit your enemies and extend a hand of forgiveness. Create a perfect world in your visualization and just indulge in that peaceful world for a few minutes. When you are done with your meditation, you will be in the right place to let go of all your fears and anxiety. This calming effect activates the vagus nerve, allowing you to live a normal life again.

Simple Step by Step Guide to Meditation

Step1: Prepare the Meditation Room and Tools

For meditation to be successful, you must find a quiet location without interruptions. You can meditate in your bedroom or in an open space. It is important that the meditation location has plenty of fresh air and that it allows you to enjoy peace during meditation. You will also need a meditation mat or a right-back chair. You may need some meditation music, but it is not compulsory.

Step 2: Position Yourself for Meditation

Before you start your meditation, ensure that you have enough time to complete the session. Switch off all interruptions such as your cell phone and only use your watch to set a reminder for timing purposes. Position yourself on the mat in a sitting posture with your legs right in front. Sit in an upright position and allow yourself to freely breathe in the fresh air.

If you are using a chair, ensure your back is aligned parallel to the straight back of the chair. This allows your back to be in an upright position, which is perfect for free breathing.

Step 3: Close Your Eyes and Focus on Your Breath

To prepare your mind for meditation, you need to draw your concentration. The easiest way to start concentrating is by focusing on your breathing for about 5 minutes. Do not try controlling how you breathe. Just focus your thoughts on it and feel how the air goes in and comes out. This will raise your awareness of the environment and will allow you to concentrate on the moment.

Step 4: Get into Visualization

Once your mind has been prepared for the process, get deep into visualization. With any type of meditation, you can follow this process. You only start by preparing your room, position yourself, and prepare your mind. Once you are ready, you can now focus your mind on whatever it is that the meditation technique requires. For instance, in focused meditation, you may now open your eyes and choose to focus on the ceiling in the room. If you know that you will be performing focused meditation, ensure that there is something you can focus on in the room. Interestingly, you cannot lack something to look at and try to describe in your own understanding. If you are performing peace, love, and kindness meditation, you have to close your eyes and create the images in your head. You have to start visualizing your activities as the ambassador for peace to those who need it. It is much simple if you close your eyes and only focus on the meditation for a given period of time.

Natural Ways of Vagus Nerve Stimulation

Besides meditation, slow breathing, and yoga, there are other techniques of vagus nerve stimulation that are less harmful.

Look at these techniques and use them to stimulate your vagus nerve when you are anxious or nervous.

Chewing Gum: Chewing gum leads to the secretion of CCK, a gut hormone that directly activates vagal impulses. This explains why people are likely to remain active for long hours while chewing gum. When a person chews gum, he/she can go for hours without taking food. This is due to the vagal impulses that CCK sends to the brain. The brain is tricked into thinking that the person is eating food. This trick can be used to reduce the sensory actions that lead to feelings of hunger in a person.

Eat High Fiber Foods: High fiber foods have also been found to be helpful in stimulating the action of the vagus nerve. Fiber foods are a good source of GLP-1, a satiating hormone that is responsible for the stimulating vagus impulses in the brain. This hormone helps slow down gut action and as a result, makes a person feel fuller for a long time. Some of the important high fiber foods include grains such as barley and peas. You can also rely on carrots, nuts, and potatoes, among others.

Tai Chi: We have already looked at tai-chi as one of the most effective ways of stimulating the vagus nerve. This is a 100% natural process since it does not involve the use of electronic gadgets. Tai-chi is known for its ability to increase heart rate variability; as a result, directly influencing the actions of the vagus nerve.

Gargling: Gargling may seem like child's play to many, but it is an important exercise that may influence your vagus nerve health. Gargling activates the vagus nerve and stimulates the gastrointestinal tract. Naturally, it is the vagus nerve that is supposed to activate the muscles behind the throat, allowing you to gargle. However, in a case where the action of the vagus nerve is slow, and the body needs some stimulation, self-induced gargling leads to the contraction of the muscles in the back of your throat, hence stimulating the vagus nerve. You can naturally stimulate your vagus nerve by gargling water before you swallow it.

Singing or Chanting: Another way of influencing the activity of your vagus nerve us through singing and chanting. Singing increases heart variability, just like it is the case with tai chi. Some of the best chants and songs include humming, mantra recitation, hymn singing, etc. These types of songs or any hyperactivity dance and song performance can influence your vagus nerve to a large extent. When you sing, you stimulate the vagus pump, which sends relaxing waves to the brain through the choir. If you chant or sing at the top of your voice, you activate the muscles behind the throat, which stimulate the vagus nerve for action.

Conclusion

You do not want to live your life wrestling with depression and anxiety, or grappling with stomach issues. Ultimately, one of the best methods of treatment is through the use of the vagus nerve. In using the vagus nerve, you are able to treat these issues at home. In being at home and stimulating the vagus nerve, you not only save money and time, but you also take the power back into your own hands. No longer are you dependent upon someone or something else to keep your body functioning—you can do it yourself. No longer do you feel like you have to keep going to appointment after appointment with no luck—you may be able to treat your problems with the vagus nerve and stimulating it, allowing instead for that time to be better spent doing other, more meaningful things, such as spending it with your children.

After reading this, the next natural line of action for you is to begin to experiment. Which of the methods included work best for you? Which do not seem to work well at all? Remember, every person is different, and everyone will respond to the same situation differently. However, keep in mind that these methods should be attempted two or three times before you truly give up on them. Just because you had little success the first time does not mean that the same method will fail you again if you try it again. Experiment around with all of the methods that have been given to you and see which you like.

Of course, you may also choose to seek out alternative methods to treat yourself as well. You may choose to treat yourself with other techniques and methods, such as using medication, and that is okay, too. Ultimately, this book existed to be your guide to the vagus nerve. It sought to make sure that you had all of the necessary information to make an informed decision on how to address your own issues, and if you have done that, then this book has done its job.

Remember, no matter how you are suffering, you do not have to. There is no reason for you to live your life in suffering. You should be able to live your life happily, healthily, and pain-free. If this means that you are meditating daily, then so be it. Ultimately, you will find a method that will work well for you, and when you do, you will not want to let it go—for good reason.

Good luck to you on your journey toward wellness. No matter whether you choose to continue to use the vagus nerve or choose other methods, you deserve the health and wellness that is waiting for you on the other side. All you need to do is figure out exactly how to get it, and you will find that it is attainable once and for all.